FRACTURES, DIS-LO-CA-TIONS, AND SPRAINS

FRACTURES, DIS-LO-CA-TIONS, AND SPRAINS

ALAN E. NOURSE

A FIRST BOOK | FRANKLIN WATTS | NEW YORK | LONDON | 1978

Photographs courtesy of the Denver Museum of Natural History: p. 6; SCALA/EPA: pp. 8 (top and bottom), 10, and 22; and Jacob F. Katz, M.D., Mount Sinai School of Medicine of the City University of New York: p. 26.

Library of Congress Cataloging in Publication Data

Nourse, Alan Edward.
Fractures, dislocations, and sprains.

(A First book)
Bibliography: p.
Includes index.
SUMMARY: Discusses bones and joint structures, the fractures, dislocations, and sprains that injure them, and techniques of treatment, including first aid.
1. Fractures—Juvenile literature. 2. Dislocations—Juvenile literature. 3. Sprains—Juvenile literature. [1. Fractures. 2. Dislocations. 3. Sprains] I. Title.
RD101.N68 617'.1 78-6855
ISBN 0-531-01494-0

Diagrams by Rod Slater

Printed in the United States of America
5 4

CONTENTS

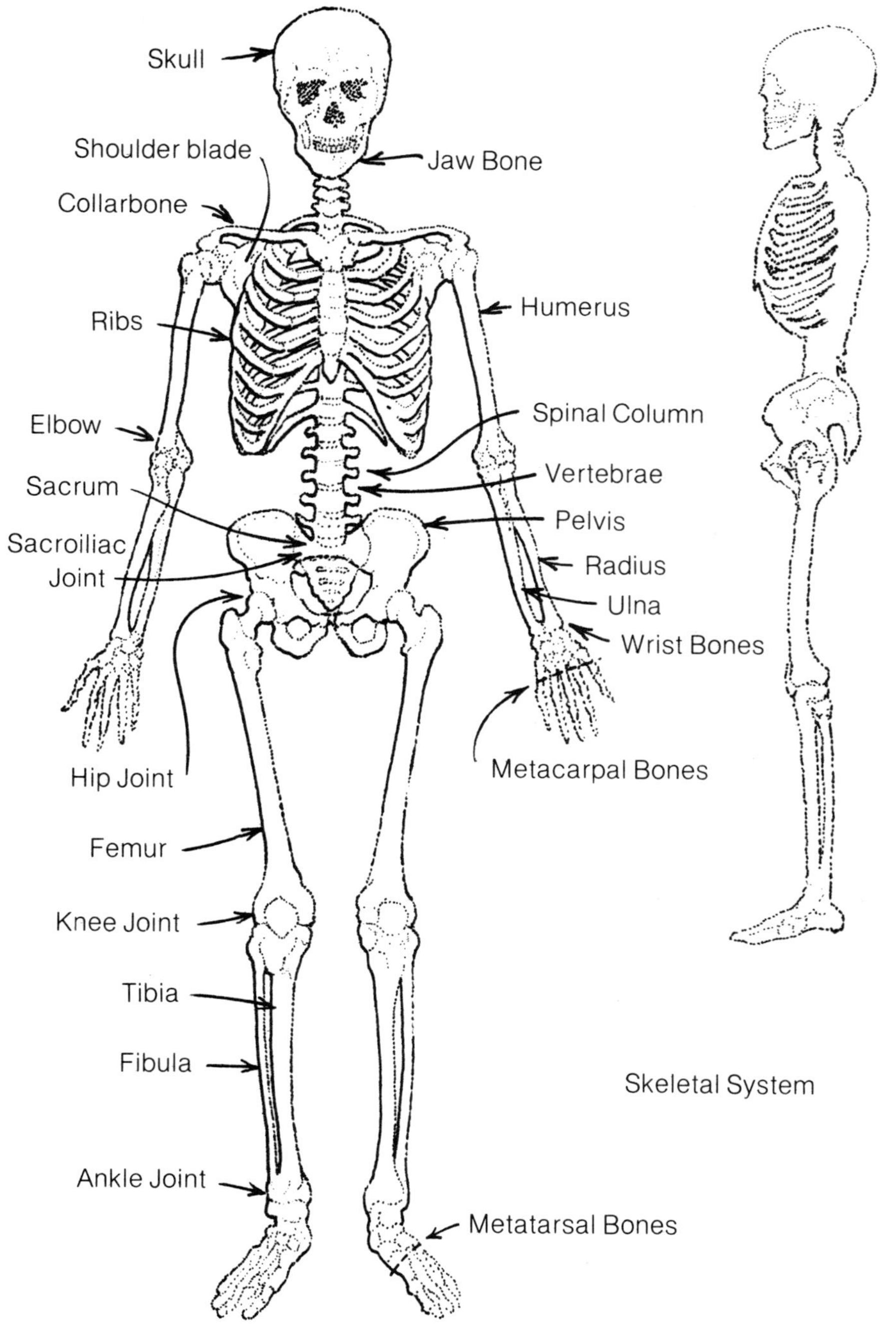

Skeletal System

CHAPTER 1
ACCIDENTS AND INJURIES

The snow on the ski slopes is the best it's been all winter. You've been skiing since nine in the morning, hardly even stopping for lunch. Now it's almost four o'clock, and there's time for just one last run before the bus leaves for home.

You and your friend start down the slope, crisscrossing in front of each other and making fancy turns. Then, without warning, a stranger comes down, fast, on a collision course. At the last moment you swing aside—and then you are flying head over heels, landing with a crash. You think you hear a loud popping sound as you strike, and you try to roll over to look at your skis.

You don't roll far. The skis are fine, but your lower leg is not. There is a cutting pain just below the right knee, and your right foot seems to be turned in the wrong direction.

You suddenly realize your leg is broken, and that this is the end of your skiing season. And you are right. You have broken your right tibia, the large bone in the lower leg. It will be a matter of five to six months before that bone heals completely —perhaps in time for hiking next summer.

It is your first football game of the season, and you and your teammates are in top shape and ready to go. You have high hopes of winning, but the opposing team is fast and hard-hitting. At halftime, you are trailing by a touchdown, and you need another score badly. The opportunity comes when the other team fumbles deep in their own territory, and you fall on the ball.

Unfortunately, ten other players fall on *you*—and when you try to get up, you have severe pain in your shoulder and find that you can't move your arm. In fact, the arm seems to be hanging in the wrong position altogether, and as your teammates help you off the field you're sure that you've broken it.

Not so, the doctor tells you in the Emergency Room half an hour later. No bones are broken—but the blow you received in the scramble dislocated your shoulder. The rounded upper end of the humerus bone—the large bone of the upper arm—was wrenched out of its normal place in the shoulder socket. After giving you some medicine to help relieve the pain and muscle cramping, the doctor has you lie face down on a wheeled stretcher with your arm hanging free over one edge. And after some pulling and tugging, the bone slips back again into the proper position in the shoulder. The moment it does, the pain in the shoulder stops. Though you can again move your arm, the doctor insists upon wrapping it tightly against your chest. It will be several weeks before you can return to full normal use of that arm—not as long as it takes a broken bone to heal, but long enough to keep you off the football field for the rest of the season.

You are near the end of a long day of summer hiking, coming down from one of the high lakes where you and your family have been fishing. It is late, and you still have 2 miles (3.2 km) of rough trail down to the parking lot, so you try to hurry, neglecting to stop and rest even though your legs feel very tired and unstable.

Suddenly you catch a toe under a root and go down, wrenching your ankle severely. It hurts so badly you can't put any weight on it. You take off your boot and soak your ankle in the cold water of the creek nearby, but it seems to be swelling just the same.

Finally, your family gets the ankle wrapped tightly with an Ace bandage, and you force your boot back on again. By hobbling, you can make your way on down, but, by the time you reach the car, your ankle is so painful you can hardly bear to touch foot to ground. Later that evening in the doctor's office, your whole ankle is swollen and purple and extremely tender, but you learn that no bone is broken, nor is there any joint dislocation. You have merely sprained the ankle, tearing part of the tough layer of fibrous tissue that supports the ankle joint. For two days you are stuck in bed, with your ankle wrapped snugly and your whole foot elevated on a couple of pillows. Because of the severity of the sprain, you will have to use crutches to get around for two or three weeks, and it may be another month or more before your ankle recovers full strength.

Fractures. Dislocations. Sprains. All three are serious injuries. All three happen often to active young people. All three involve the bones and joints of the body. All are painful, and all seem to take almost forever to heal.

It's no wonder active young people hate these injuries so much. Anybody can put up with a head cold or a cut finger or even a case of flu. Such things are over in a week or so. But the healing of fractures, dislocations, and sprains can drag on for days and weeks and months. What's more, there is nothing you can do to speed up the healing, and if you get impatient and try to use the injured bone or joint before it is ready to be used, you are very likely to cause even more damage than before.

These injuries often result from sporting activities, and they happen very frequently. If you have not yet had a fracture, dislocation, or sprain, you can be pretty sure your turn is coming. Therefore, it is important to have some idea of what these injuries are and why they occur, of why they take so long to heal and why proper healing is so important.

To understand these things, we must start at the beginning. Let's take a brief look at the special kinds of body structures involved in these injuries—bone, cartilage, and joint structures, and the tendons and ligaments that help to hold the joints together.

CHAPTER 2

BONES AND JOINTS ALIVE

Of all the tissues in the body, none is more important to our shape, strength, and activity than our bones. (A tissue is any group of cells that forms a part of the body.) Imagine for a moment a Joe Namath on the football field without any bones! Or a Chris Evert on the tennis court, or a Muhammad Ali in the boxing ring! Without bones to shape and hold up their bodies, they would be nothing but lumps of twitching muscle.

It is bone that allows you to stand erect and gives your body its shape: the rounded head, the shoulders and chest, the two movable arms, and the legs that allow you to walk, run, jump, or stand on tiptoe.

You may never have seen living bone. Of course you've seen chunks of bone in a beef pot roast or a leg of lamb. But these are only fragments of animal bones that are no longer living. You may have seen a deer skull in the woods, or the

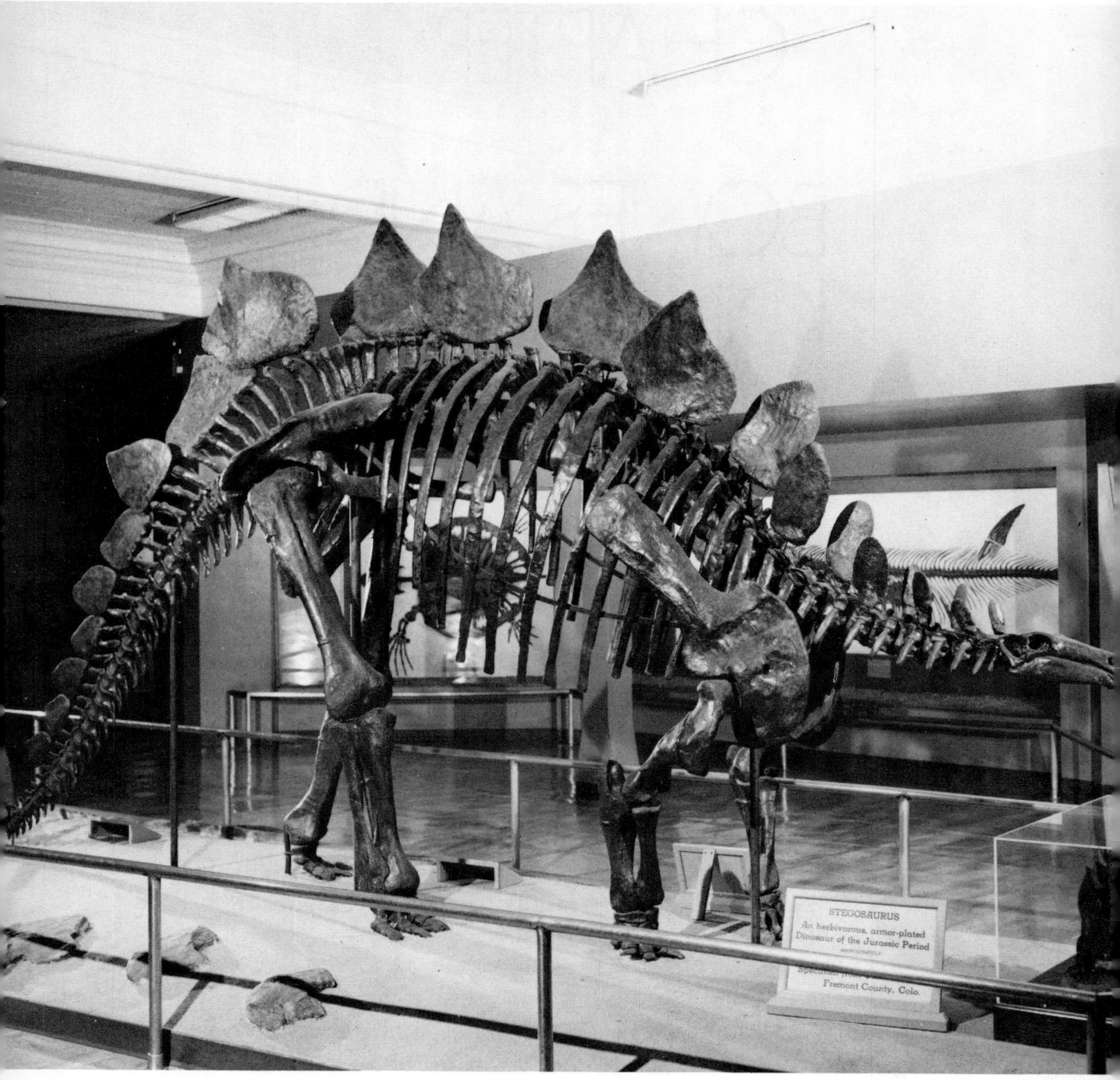
STEGOSAURUS
An herbivorous, armor-plated
Dinosaur of the Jurassic Period
Fremont County, Colo.

put-together bones of a prehistoric dinosaur in a museum. If so, you may have realized that dead bone (along with teeth) is one of the most durable substances in the world. Human bones as much as ten thousand years old have been discovered in parts of Africa, and the five-thousand-year-old bones of Egyptian kings have been preserved almost as well as if their owners had died just last year.

A PICTURE OF LIVING BONE

The bone in our body differs from the dead bone in an Egyptian mummy in one important way: it is very much alive—as much as any other structure in the body. Living bone is made up of a microscopic network of living cells in which insoluble calcium and phosphoric chemicals have been laid down, like cement, to give the bone its special hardness. By way of blood vessels blood enters and leaves the bone so that oxygen can reach all the bone cells and carbon dioxide and waste materials can be carried away. True, the cells in bone are not as active as are the cells in our skin or muscles. And the blood supply to bone is not very good either. Thus, bone heals very slowly when it is damaged—but heal it does, just like any other living tissue.

There are two major kinds of bone tissue, both often found working together in the same bone. In a leg bone, for example, the long, narrow shaft is made of a very dense, hard, bony material. It is built like a hollow tube, which makes it both amazingly light and amazingly strong. This is important to a long-distance runner, whose legs must absorb several

A put-together skeleton of the dinosaur Stegosaurus.

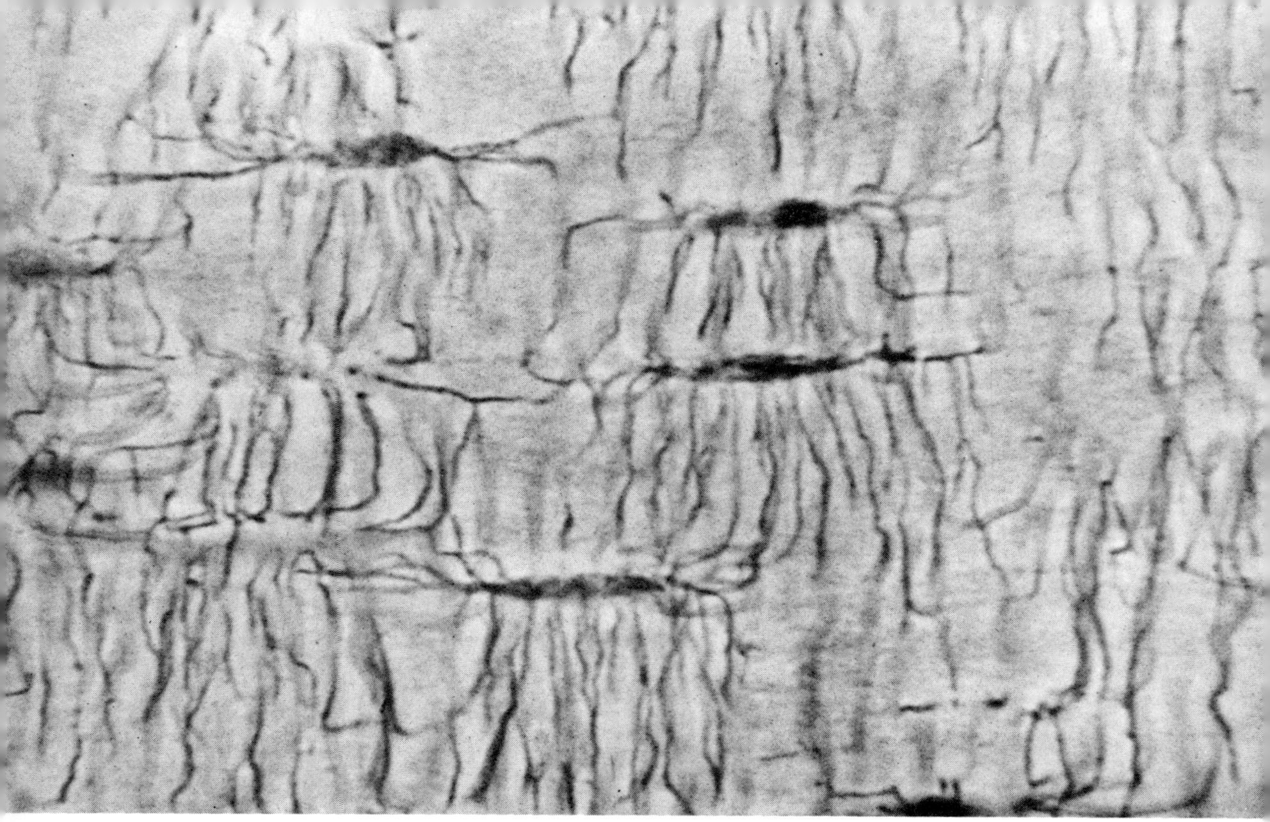

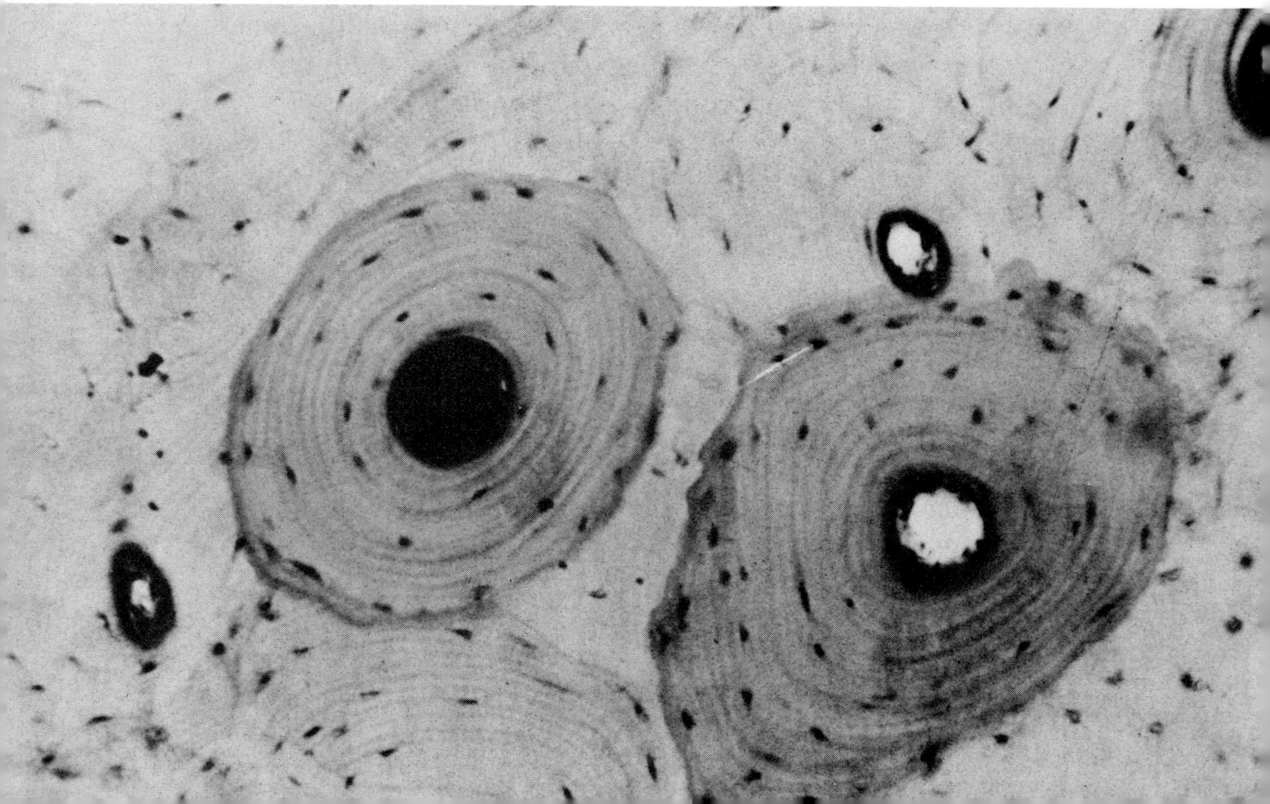

hundred pounds (kilograms) of weight each time his or her foot hits the ground. It is even more important to the pole vaulter, whose leg bones may have to absorb much, much more pressure on hitting the ground after a 12-foot (3.5-m) vault.

The ends of the leg bones, however, are built in a different way. They tend to bulge out and are covered all over with a layer of hard, dense bone. But their interior is filled with a spongy bone that has a very rich blood supply. This spongy bone looks soft and weak, but it is built with special "strength lines," like reinforcing bars in concrete, to make it strong. All in all, few substances other than steel are stronger than living bone. Yet the total weight of all of the bone in your body is probably less than 30 pounds (13.5 kg). Steel bars and tubes of equal shape and strength would weigh ten times as much.

However, bone must do far more than provide shape and support for the body. It must also provide us a means for moving about. Thus, the bones of the arms, wrists, hands, legs, ankles, feet, chest, and back all fit together to form many different kinds of connections, or joints. These joints permit motion where it is necessary and prevent it where it would be dangerous. It is the muscles attached to the bone across these joints which permit us to move. In most cases, the joint muscles work in opposite pairs. When one muscle of such a pair tightens or *contracts* and pulls on a bone, the opposite muscle *relaxes* and allows the bone to move. Then,

Above, living bone cells. Below, a cross section of hard, living bone.

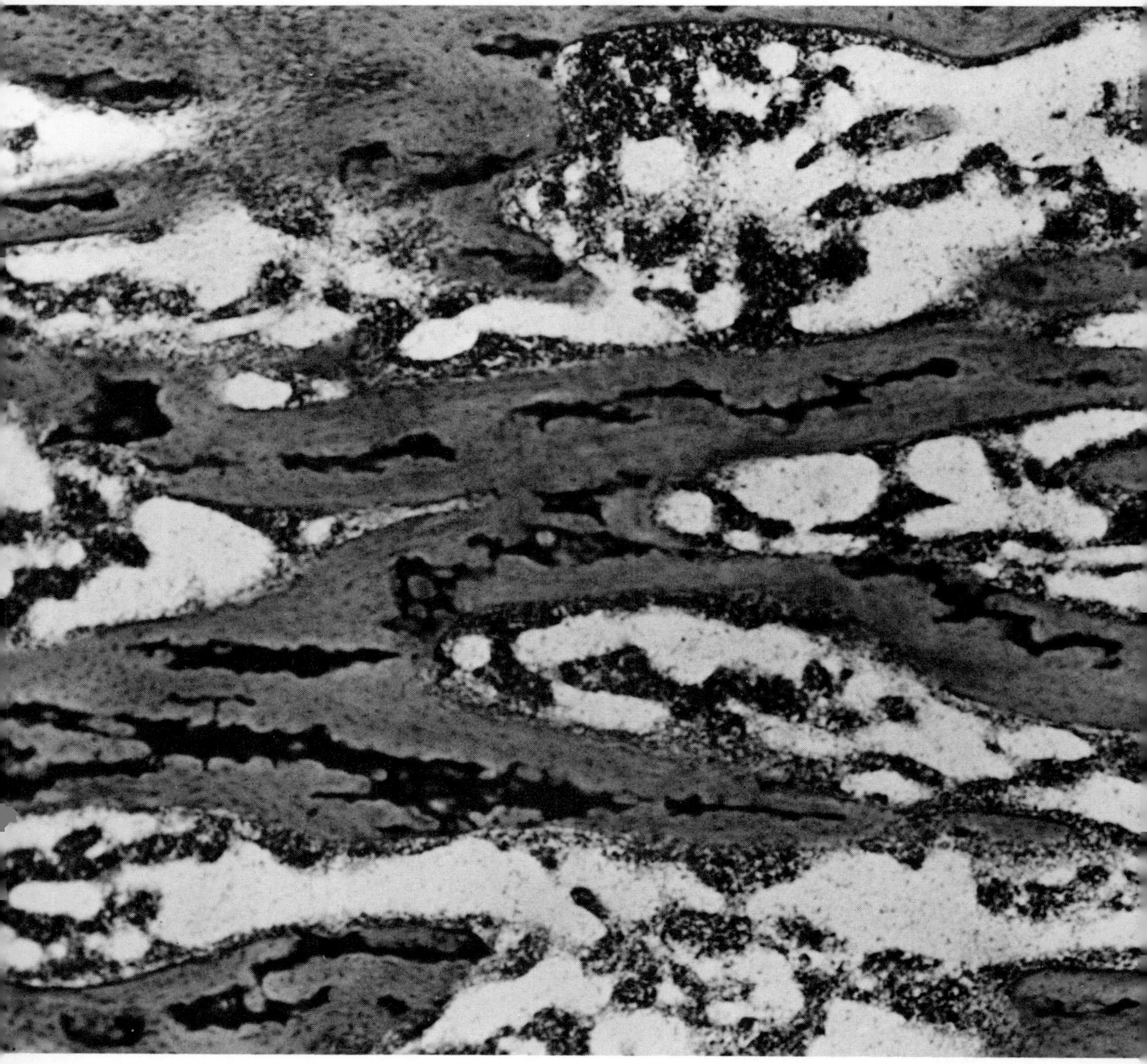

when the opposite muscle contracts and pulls the bone back again, the first muscle relaxes.

To see how this works, hold your arm out straight from your shoulder with your palm up. Now raise your forearm up to a right angle at your elbow. What makes the forearm lift up? The answer is, the heavy muscle called the biceps on the inner surface of the upper arm. This muscle has contracted across the elbow joint and lifted the bones of the forearm. You can feel that the biceps muscle is bulging and much shorter than it was when the arm was extended out straight. Now straighten the arm out again and feel the biceps muscle. You'll see that it is much longer and feels flabby—but now the triceps muscle on the back of the upper arm (opposite the biceps) feels bulging and tight. One muscle tightens or contracts while the other relaxes, and vice versa. It is the two muscles working as a team in this manner that allows you to bend and straighten your elbow.

It is the same with other movable joints. Each of your finger bones, for example, is connected by means of a pair of long, stringlike tendons to muscles in your forearm. (A tendon is a tough, strong tissue, much like a narrow leather shoestring, which binds muscle to bone.) When the muscles on the back of your arm contract, their tendons pull your fingers out straight or *extend* them; these muscles are known as finger extenders. Their opposite muscles on the inner surface of the forearm are called finger flexors because when they contract, their tendons bend or *flex* the fingers in toward the palm.

Spongy bone.

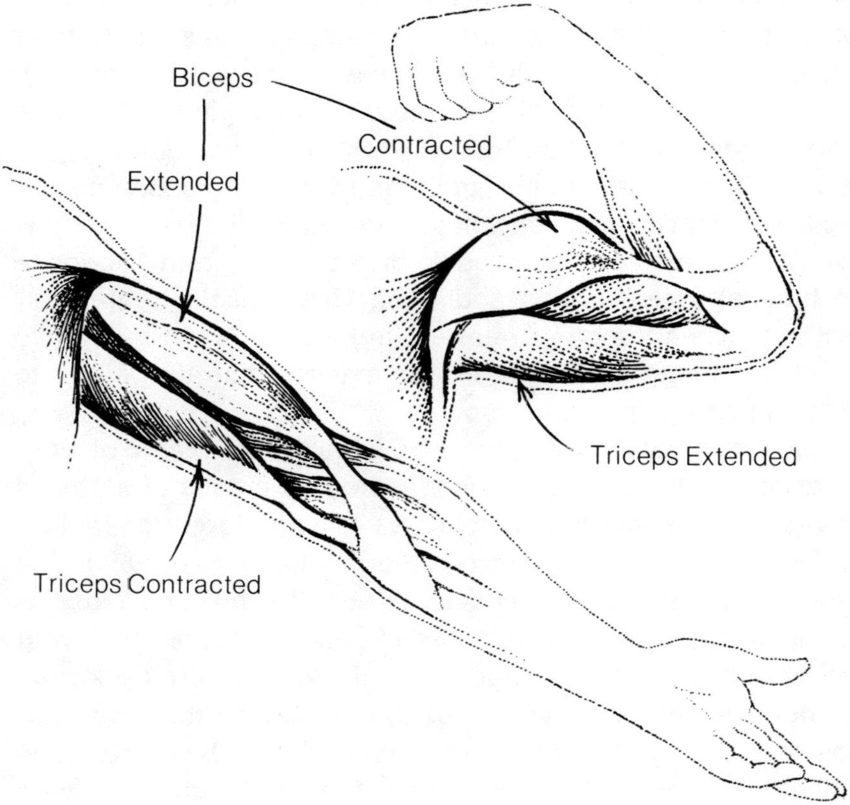
Biceps
Contracted
Extended
Triceps Extended
Triceps Contracted

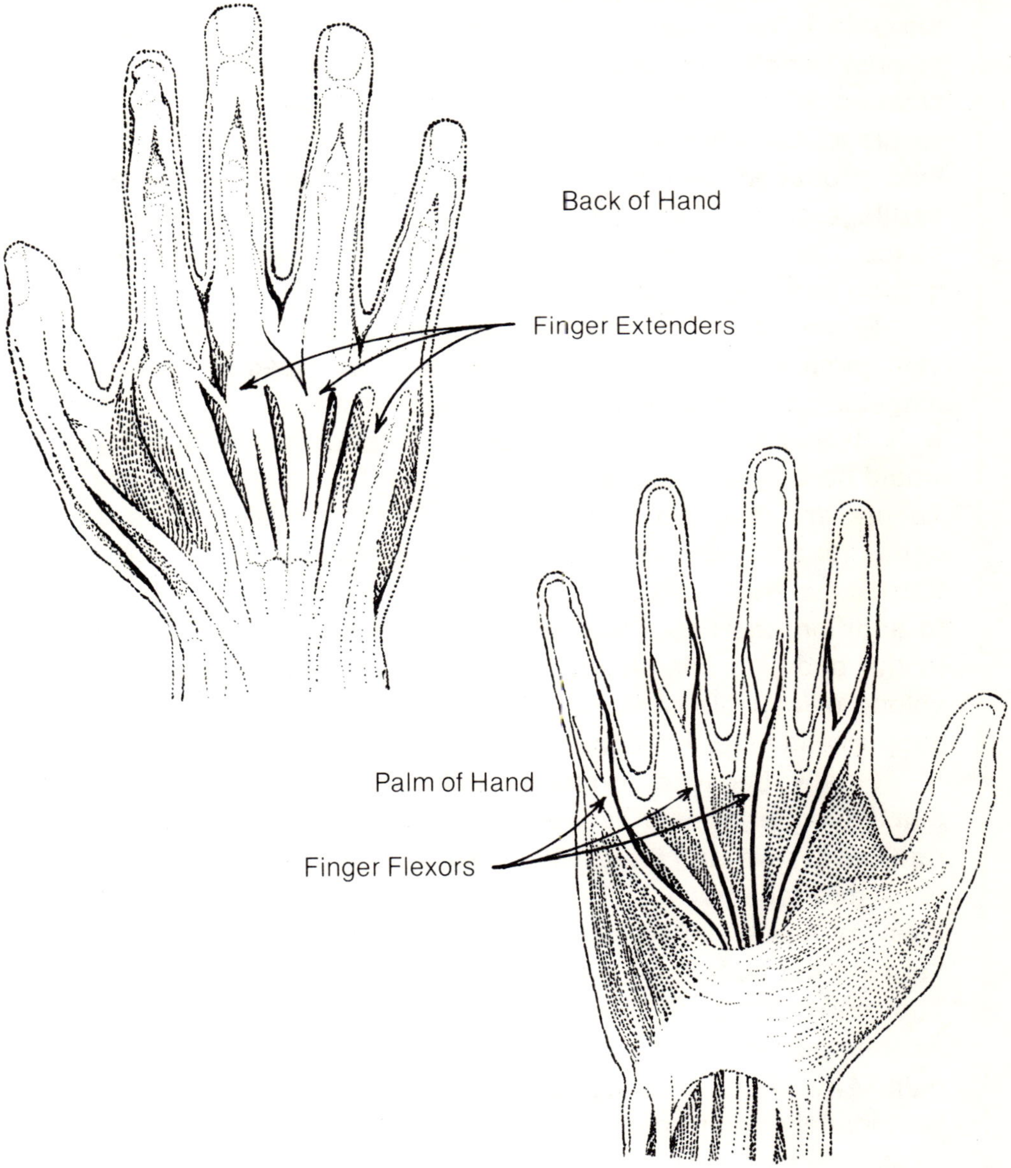
Back of Hand
Finger Extenders
Palm of Hand
Finger Flexors

When the ends of bones move against each other at the movable joints, why don't we feel a rough grating of bone against bone? The reason is that these fitted bone ends are covered with a soft, smooth variation of bony tissue called cartilage. Cartilage is kept smooth and slippery by a sticky fluid produced by the joints. This fluid actually makes the cartilage covering the bone ends about ten times as slippery as ice. Under normal conditions, the joints move without any grating or friction at all.

Some joints not only permit some motion but also prevent motion that might be dangerous. We need a smooth, hingelike motion of the knee joint, for example, in order to walk. If that same joint were able to twist or rotate, our legs would be very unstable and we would be forever falling down. To prevent this, the knee joint contains special chunks of cartilage and additional strong ligaments—strips of tough fibrous material—to keep the knee from rotating or wobbling. In addition, the knee (like all the other major movable joints in the body) is completely surrounded by a tight-fitting envelope or capsule of fibrous tissue which provides additional support and helps keep the joint from coming unhinged.

Finally, because an injured or broken bone can severely damage softer structures around it if we don't treat it properly right away, we are fitted with a kind of "early warning system" that tells us when something has happened to bone. A layer of tissue called periosteum (a medical term meaning "around the bone") is stretched over the outside of the bone. The periosteum contains many blood vessels and—even more important—a thick network of nerve fibers sensitive to pain. Any injury or bruising of this sensitive bone covering immediately sends pain signals flashing to the brain, telling us at once that something has gone wrong.

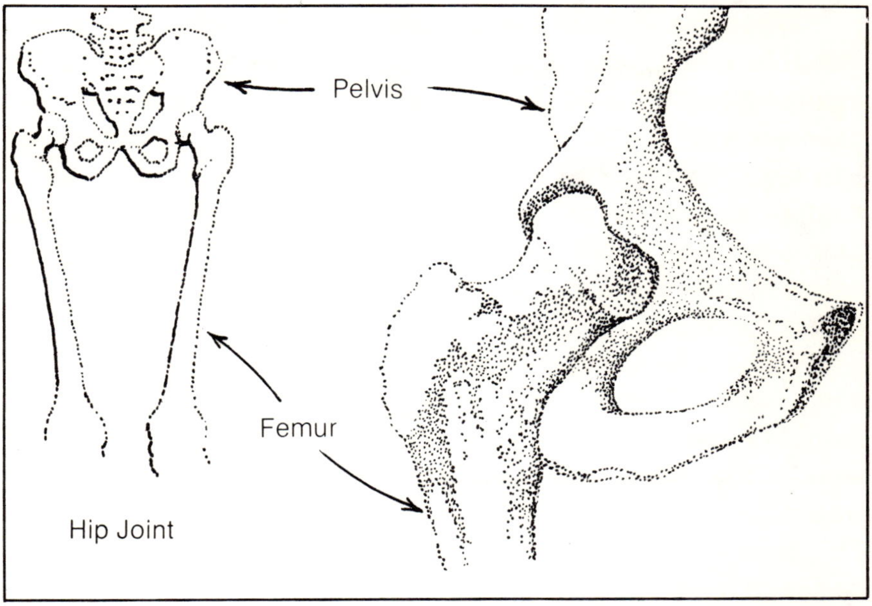

MORE ABOUT JOINTS

At the knee, a simple hinge joint is all that is needed. But the joint that connects the upper end of the femur, or thigh bone, with the saddlelike pelvis is more complicated. This so-called "hip joint" must carry half the weight of the body whenever we are standing up and two to three times the entire weight of the body alternately with the other hip joint whenever we walk or run. It must also allow circular or rotary motion so that we can rotate our entire leg outward to a certain degree or in toward the other leg to a certain degree, lift it up in front of us or move it back behind us. To accomplish this, a large spur at the upper end of the thighbone ends in a rounded ball, and the matching pelvic bone has a

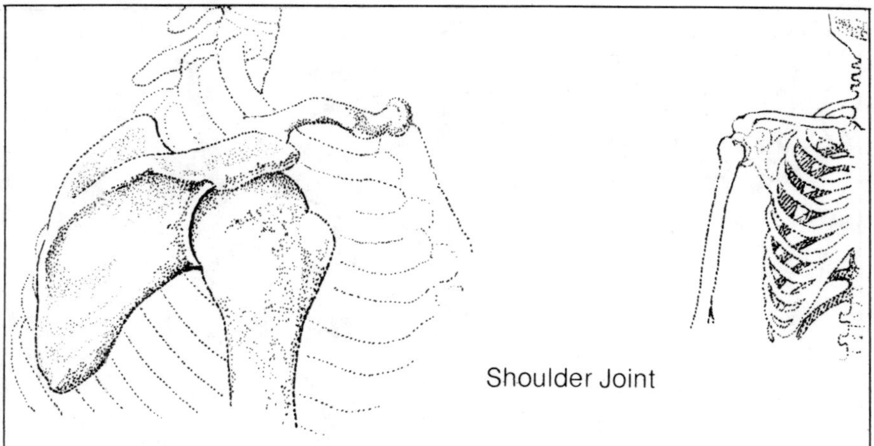

Shoulder Joint

deep circular socket into which this ball fits. It is this ball-and-socket arrangement that permits the hip joint to carry heavy weights for long periods of time as well as allow the leg to move in more different directions than the knee.

The shoulder joint is another ball-and-socket joint. But, here, strength and the ability to bear weight are less important than allowing for a high degree of circular or rotary arm motion. Thus, in the shoulder, the ball-and-socket joint is much shallower. This allows greater movement and agility of the shoulder but less strength for weight-bearing. And because the shallow ball-and-socket joint of the shoulder is fairly weak, it can sometimes be jarred out of place, or dislocated.

Other joints have special points of interest. Like the knee joint, the joints between the small bones of the fingers are simple hinge joints. Any attempts to twist or rotate these joints will cause discomfort. The thumb, however, can rotate at its joint with the wrist bones enough to bend the thumb around and touch the fingertips. Many scientists believe that the ability of very primitive humans to rotate their thumbs allowed them a tight grip on weapons or tools and was important in putting their rapidly increasing intelligence to work.

The elbow is also a hinge joint, but a very special one. Three bones are jointed at the elbow: the lower end of the upper arm bone, or humerus, connects with the two long bones in the forearm, the ulna (which you can feel as the "point of the elbow" and which extends down to form another easily felt lump above the wrist on the little finger side of the forearm) and the radius (which forms a smaller lump above the wrist on the thumb side of the forearm). The joint between the ulna and the humerus is a straightforward hinge joint that allows the forearm to move up and down. The radius, on the other hand, *rotates* at its connection with the humerus, and, by actually crisscrossing the ulna, it allows you to turn your palm either up or down.

The two upper vertebrae bones connecting the skull to the spine form another rotating joint. Working together, they allow you to turn your head from side to side (as when you shake your head "No") or to tip it up and down (as when you nod your head "Yes").

Some joints permit only a very small amount of motion. The column of vertebrae which makes up the neck and backbone must support the weight of the body and protect the spinal cord. Not much movement can be permitted here. But there is just enough movement between each of these individual bones to make it possible for you to twist your body to the right or left or to allow you to bend your back forward or (to

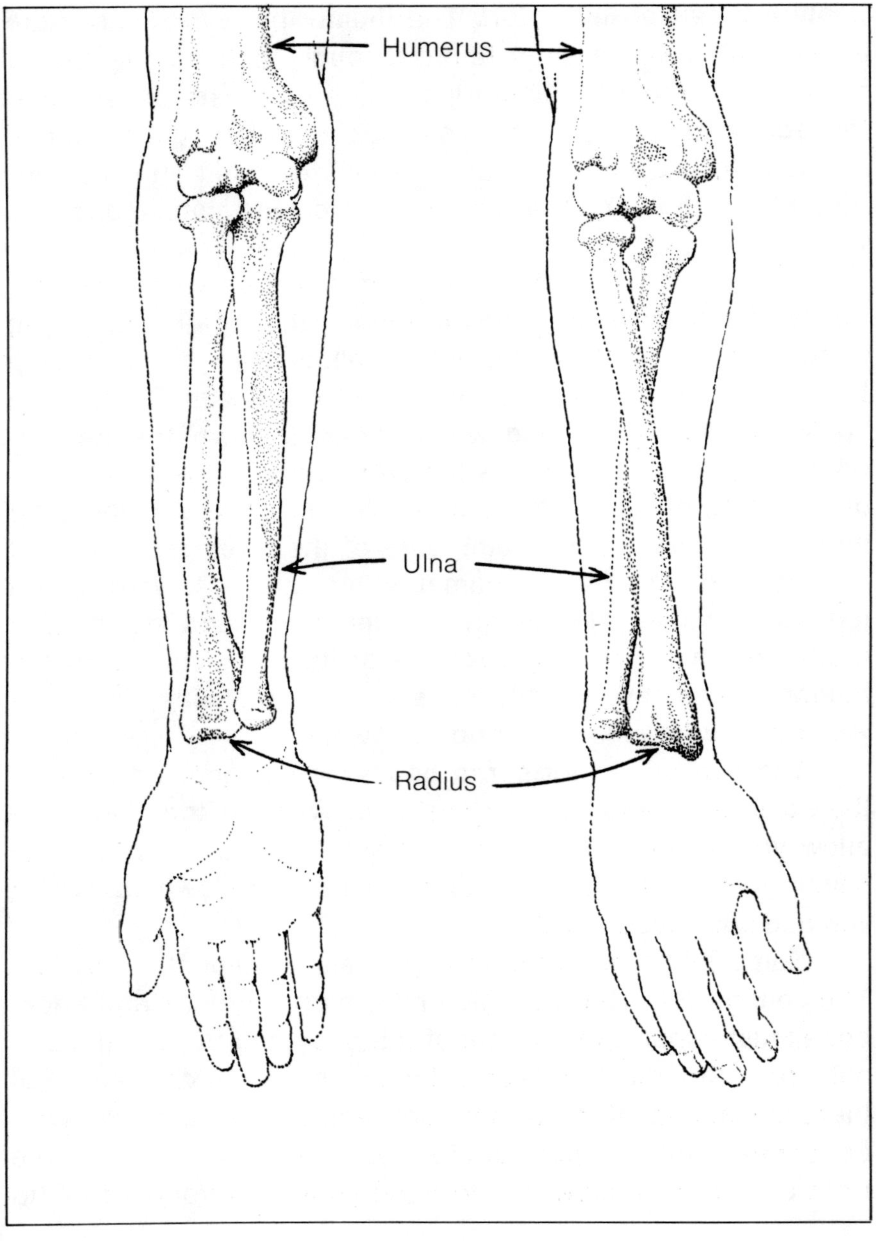
Humerus
Ulna
Radius

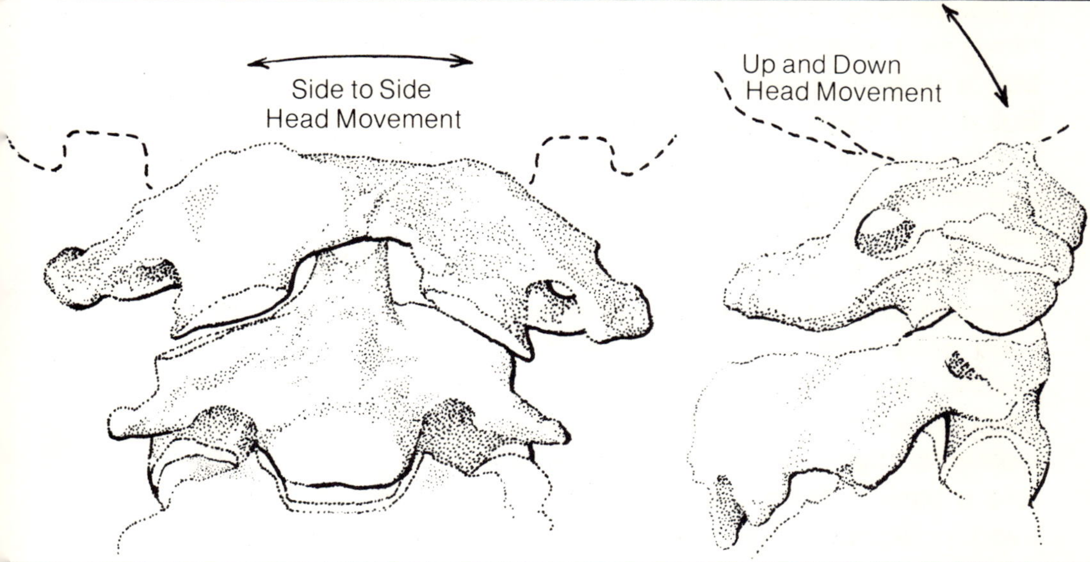
Side to Side
Head Movement
Up and Down
Head Movement

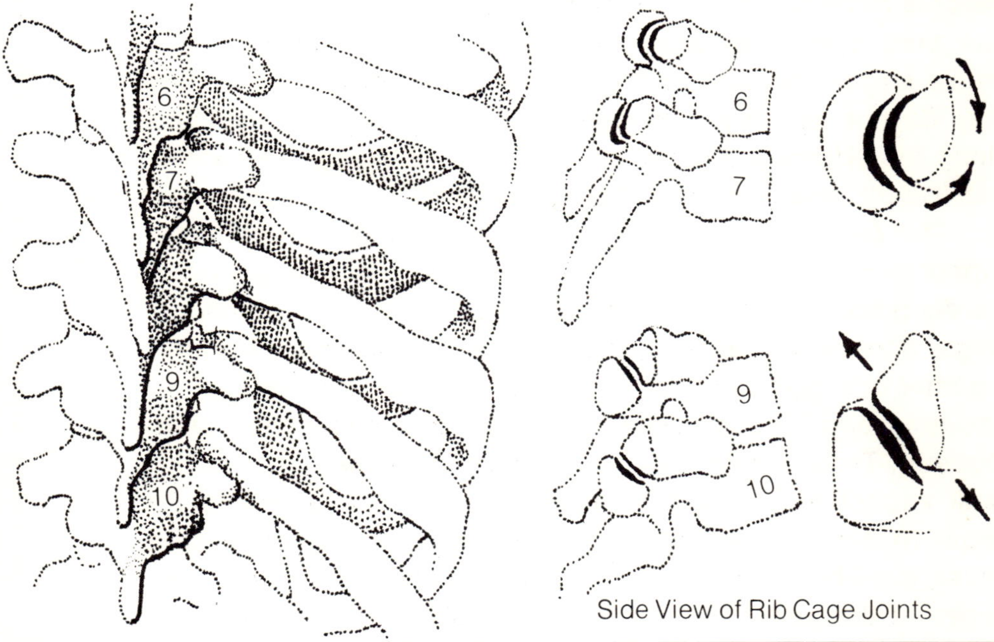
6
7
9
10
6
7
9
10
Side View of Rib Cage Joints

a smaller degree) backward. The ribs must also be able to move very slightly. We need the curved, flattened, hard rib bones to form a strong cage to protect our heart and lungs. But if that cage were completely rigid, we couldn't expand our lungs properly when breathing. Thus, there are tiny ball-and-socket joints where our ribs attach to the vertebrae, allowing the ribs to lift and fall with our breathing movements.

Finally, there are certain joints in the body that are not intended to move at all. The skull, for example, seems to be a solid protective helmet of bone. Actually, it is made up of several curving plates of bone which are connected to each other in solid interlocking joints like jigsaw puzzle pieces, welded so tightly together that they cannot be separated. Before a baby is born, these bone plates are separate and can overlap slightly. This makes it easier on the baby's head at the time of birth. During childhood, these bones remain separate, held together by tough fibrous tissue. As the child's brain grows larger and larger, these bones also grow larger. But they do not actually join together and become firmly fixed along the edges until sometime between the ages of sixteen and twenty, when the brain has grown as large as it ever will.

The pelvis is much the same. This saddle-shaped bone supports the internal organs of the abdomen and provides the deep sockets of the hip joints. Actually, the pelvis is not a single bone at all but is made up of six bones solidly glued together into one piece. In this case, however, the "gluing" is due to strong fibrous tissue and cartilage binding the bones together. These joints are almost as solid as the joints in the skull except at one special time of life: when a woman is about to have a baby. At this time certain body chemicals cause the fibrous tissue and cartilage between some of the bones of the pelvis to loosen ever so slightly, providing just a tiny bit of give. This give allows these bones to separate slightly at the time of the child's birth, making it easier for the baby to be born. Afterward, these joints once again return to their normal solid firmness.

THE LIFE CYCLE OF BONE

You might think, from what we have said, that living bone is exactly the same whether a person is a baby, a teenager, or an eighty-year-old grandmother. Not so. In fact, bone is constantly growing and changing from the time when it first forms before birth right on through to the end of a person's life.

Bone formation begins while a new baby is still in the mother's uterus, some months before delivery. At that time all the bones are really just cartilage or membrane, soft and rubbery, with only a hint of the final shape they will take. Then, as the baby develops, bone gradually begins to form in the cartilage as calcium and phosphorus compounds are deposited there. At the same time, these bones that have begun to form also begin to grow. Bone formation and growth is the work of two very special kinds of cells that lie within the cartilage: cells called osteoblasts, or "bone makers," and other cells called osteoclasts, or "bone dissolvers."

These two kinds of cells work in close partnership. In the long bones of the arms or legs, for instance, the osteoblasts are located in the cartilage that forms the knobby ends, depositing calcium in the center of these knobs. These bone makers are also at work along special "growth lines," depositing calcium at both ends of the bone shaft and gradually pushing the cartilage at the ends of the bones farther and farther out, so that the whole bone becomes longer.

At the same time, the osteoclasts, or "bone dissolvers,"

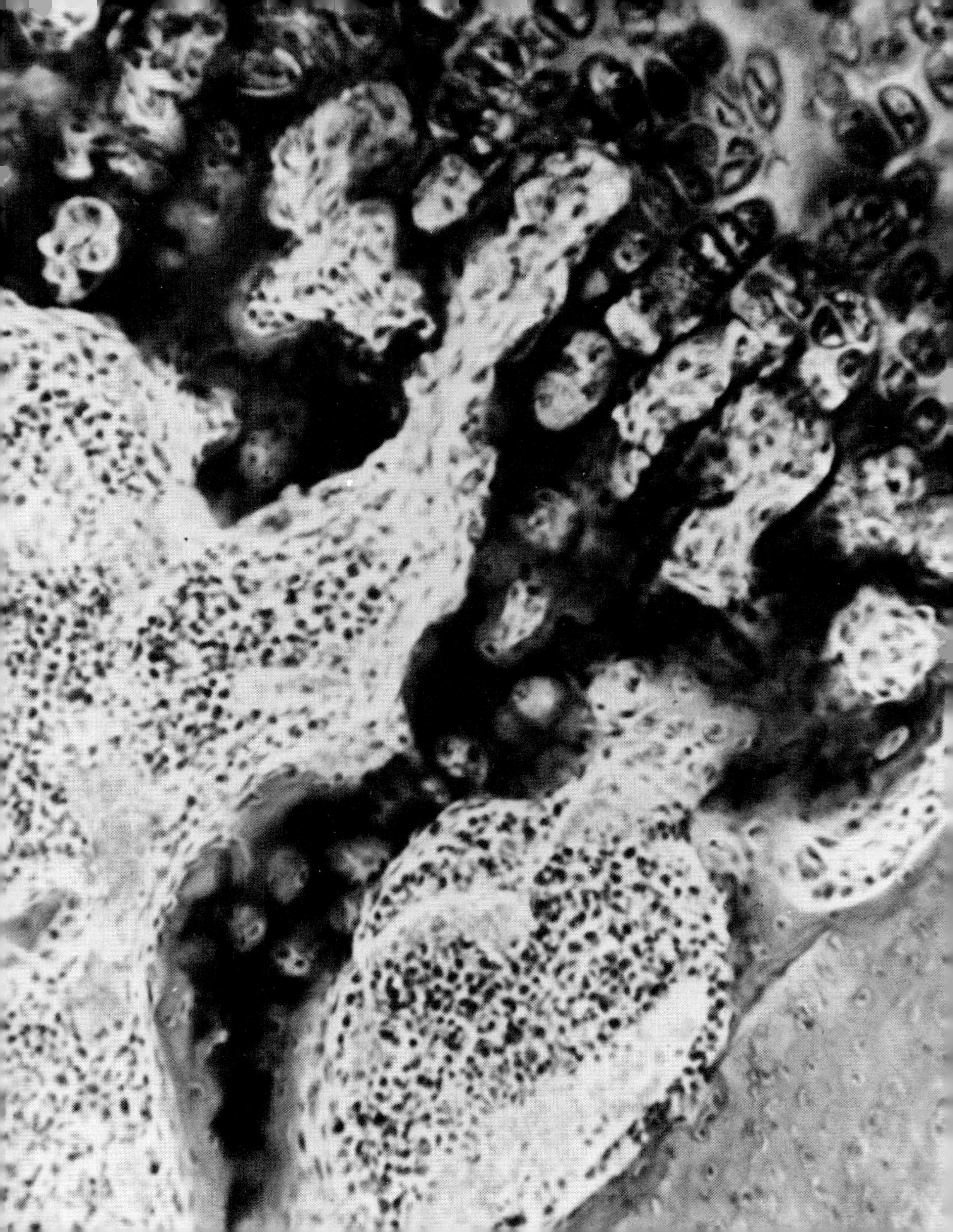

are busily dissolving bone in the center of the shafts of these long bones—hollowing them out, so to speak, but leaving the hard outer shell of the shaft for support. Eventually, the hollow shafts of these bones become filled with a fatty material known as marrow.

By the time a baby is born, the process of bone formation is well started, but the bones are still soft and rubbery, and the joints are not fully formed. During the first few years of a baby's life, these soft "baby bones" grow steadily longer, thicker, stronger and more filled with calcium. A special body chemical known as growth hormone helps set the pace for this development, but the child's diet is also important. Good supplies of protein, calcium, Vitamin C, and Vitamin D are all necessary for normal bone growth at this time of life.

By the time a child is ten or twelve years old, all of the joints will be well formed and most of the bones will have become calcified—yet X-rays still reveal a "babyish" look to the bones. The growth lines at the ends of the shafts of the long bones are still present, giving the bones an unfinished look. Then, at about age thirteen or so, the youngster—male or female—undergoes a sudden "growth spurt," becoming taller (due to a sudden increase in bone growth) and stronger (due to enlargement and strengthening of muscle). It is not until this ends—at about age fifteen for boys, somewhat earlier for girls—that the growth lines in the bone begin to disappear and the bones no longer increase in length or thickness. Whatever height you may have reached at this time will be the height you will have for the next fifty years

Bone that is developing and hardening.

of your life. Because the "growth spurt" is often not so striking in girls and levels off earlier, girls tend to be somewhat shorter than boys and have a somewhat narrower and lighter bone structure.

Just because bone stops *growing* at this time does not mean that it stops *changing.* Bit by bit, as time goes on, new bone is formed and old bone destroyed as healthy bone continually renews and replaces itself, cell by cell. By age twenty-four, all signs of growth lines will have disappeared from X-rays, and the bones will be harder and more brittle than during childhood or adolescence. While a teenager might suffer an incomplete break, or fracture, of a long bone, a man of thirty would be more likely to break the bone completely through.

Finally, with advancing age, more calcium is absorbed from the bone than is replaced. Thus, in older people bones become lighter, narrower, and more easily injured.

Even though bone is one of the toughest and strongest tissues in the body, it can be broken or fractured when the wrong kind of stress is put upon it. When a bone is fractured, it becomes totally useless until it has time enough to heal. In fact, it becomes worse than useless. A broken bone can do serious damage to surrounding tissue unless it is treated properly. Fortunately, bone has one more remarkable quality we have thus far only barely hinted at: an amazing ability to heal itself. In the next chapter we will see how bone manages to do this.

CHAPTER 3

ALL ABOUT FRACTURES

Ordinarily, we count on the strength of our bones and the smooth functioning of our joints without giving them a thought. Then something unexpected happens. We slip on the stairs, twist a leg, or fall on an outstretched arm, and things no longer work so well. But how can we tell if we have broken a bone or merely gotten a bad bruise? And if a bone *is* broken, what do we do about it?

FRACTURE OR NO FRACTURE?

Of course, not all falls or other injuries necessarily result in broken bones. If a bone *is* broken, however, we don't want to do anything to cause more damage or slow down healing. Here are some clues that can tell us if a bone is broken.

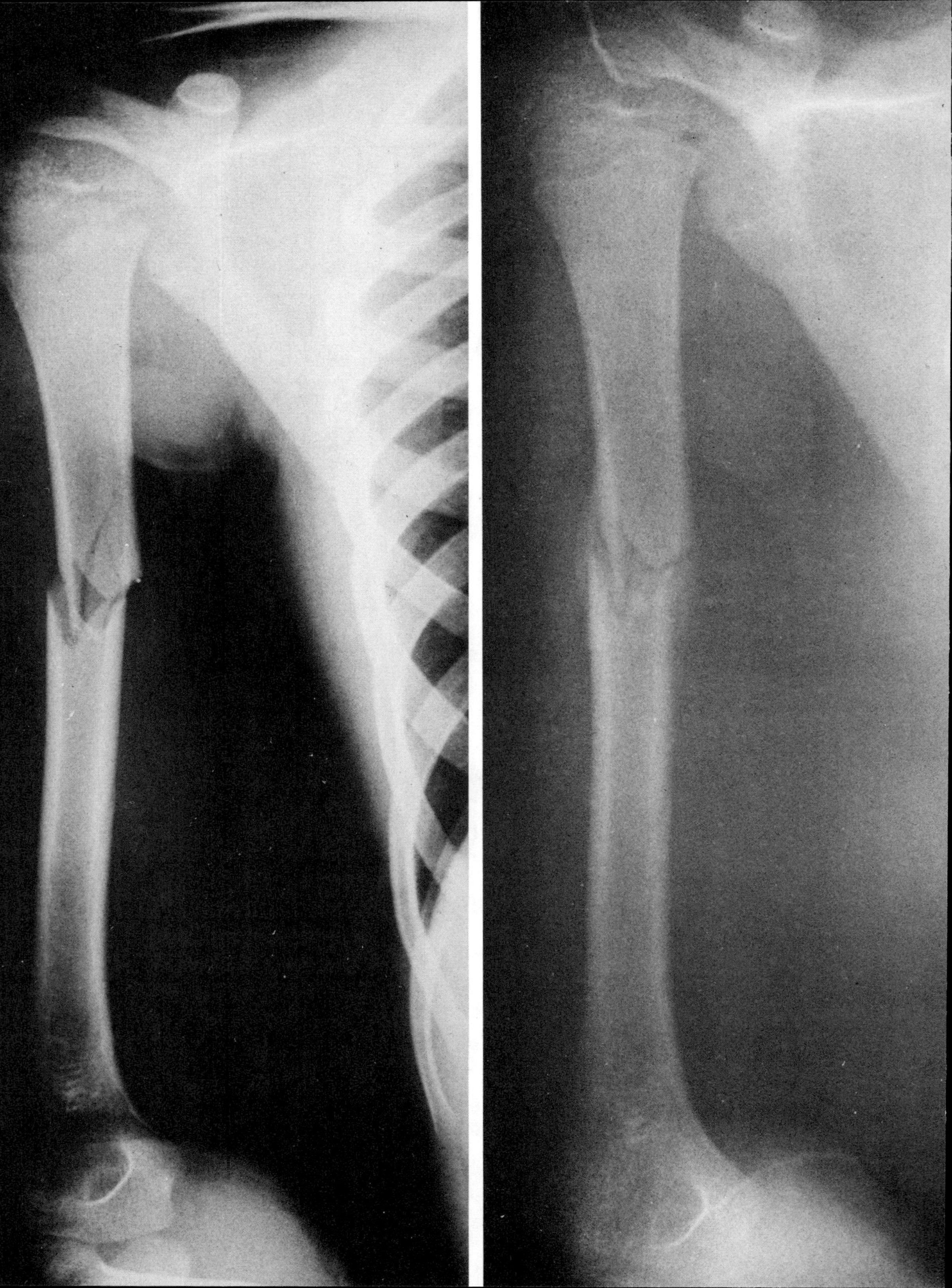

☐ *Pain.* A fractured bone almost always brings a lot of pain—not just a little pain that goes away in a few minutes but a really uncomfortable pain that stays. The pain is almost always *made worse* by any attempt to move the injured part. The pain comes from injury to the periosteum covering the bone and from cramping muscles in the area. Of course, this kind of pain *can* occur when a bone is merely bruised and not broken. But when pain is present, it's wise to assume that a fracture has occurred until proven otherwise.

☐ *Swelling.* Whenever a bone is broken, there is always bleeding from the bone itself and from surrounding muscles that have been injured. Because of this, the area around a broken bone will begin to swell up in a matter of minutes. True, such swelling might also occur from a sprain (tearing of the ligaments around a joint) or from just a severe bruise. But if the swelling occurs quickly and seems very marked and you also have continuing severe pain, you should figure the bone is probably broken until you can be certain that it isn't.

☐ *Distortion.* Since bones give our bodies "the right shape," we can often tell that a leg or arm bone has been fractured when there's something wrong with the shape of it. For instance, if you have an extremely painful forearm immediately after a fall from your bicycle, and the arm seems to have an angle where an angle shouldn't be, this is a good

Left, an X-ray of a fractured humerus, taken immediately after the injury. Right, an X-ray of the same broken humerus four weeks after the injury.

sign that you have broken a bone. A broken collarbone will often result in a hollow or depression in the upper part of the chest between the shoulder and the throat instead of the normal, smooth bulge of bone you can usually feel there.

☐ *"I heard something snap."* Bones are brittle and may pop or snap when they break. Sometimes the victim *knows* that he or she has a broken bone because of actually hearing that sound on striking the ground. Even nearby observers may hear it! If something like this happens, you'd better believe that something *did* snap, and assume that you have a broken bone until a doctor makes the final diagnosis.

FIRST AID FOR FRACTURES

Many first-aid manuals go into great detail about exactly what should be done with each individual kind of fracture that might occur. This is useful information to have. But with fast communication and modern ambulances or aid cars, it is not usually as essential as it once was. Today, when you are with someone who has suddenly broken a bone (or may have), there are just a few simple first-aid rules you should keep in mind.

First, keep the person quiet and the injured area immobile. If possible, have someone stay with the victim while someone else goes for help. Don't try to pull or tug on a broken arm or leg to "put it back into the right position." You will only cause worse pain and risk doing additional injury to the tissue around the fracture. There is a real danger, after a bone is broken, of jiggling the sharp broken bone ends so that they cut blood vessels, nerves, or muscles that were not originally injured at all. Also, such bone ends may puncture the skin, creating a wound which can then become infected.

Second, find some way to immobilize or prevent motion of the fractured area while the victim is being moved to safety. One good way to do this is to wrap the injured limb in a large, firm pillow folded lengthwise and tied in two or three places. If you don't have a pillow, use a couple of down jackets or bulky sweaters for splinting material. If the injury involves an arm or hand, wrap it in layers of bulky clothing and then pin it, splint and all, to the victim's shirt front—or with another sweater hold it close to the chest to keep it from moving. A broken finger can be splinted by placing a ball of wadded-up newspaper the size of a baseball in the victim's palm and then wrapping a shirt around it so the fingers can't move. Remember that you have two main goals: padding the injured area firmly and preventing motion. Be sure to check for warm, healthy looking skin and a pulse in the area beyond the splint, to be sure the splint is not too tight.

What if the injury seems to involve the neck or back? This is a very special, and very dangerous, kind of injury, and you really should get medical help to the scene before you do anything at all. If a bone in the neck or back is broken, careless movement of the victim can cause additional damage to the spinal cord and may even result in permanent paralysis. In most cases the best thing you can do is *keep the victim from moving at all* until help arrives. Hold the person's head steady and motionless, and prevent him or her from bending knees, hips, or shoulders. If you absolutely *must* move the person—for example, if he or she is submerged in water or is lying in some steep place in danger of falling—try to get one or two other people to help you. Working together, move the victim *flat, without rolling or twisting,* to a place of safety where he or she can be kept motionless until medical help arrives.

Using a Pillow to Protect a Fractured Arm

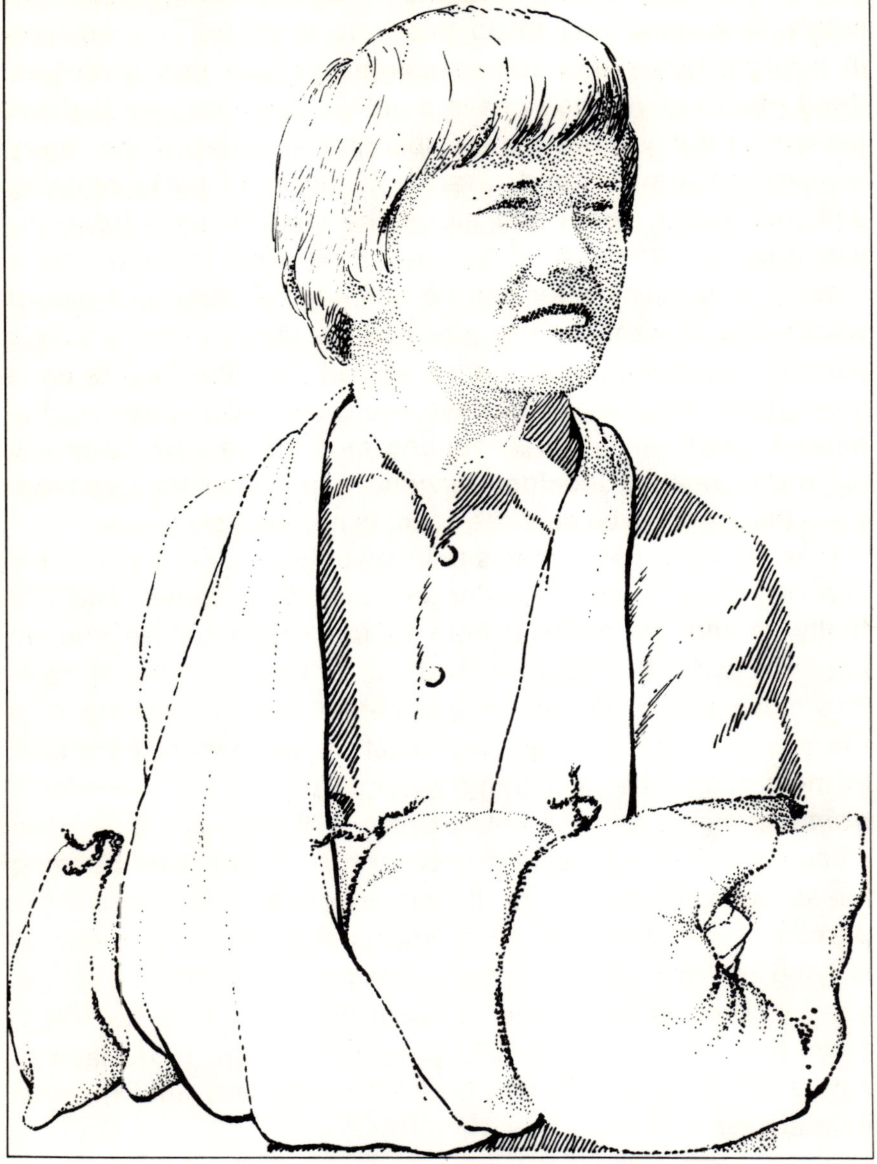

Third, pay attention to how the victim is doing. A fracture causes pain and internal bleeding. These things together can lead to a serious condition called shock. Shock is a reaction to injury in which the victim becomes shaky and faint, perspires, and feels nauseous. To help prevent this, put the victim flat on the ground with the head lower than the feet. Keep the person warm. If he or she gets sick, turn the head aside so that anything thrown up can be spit out and not accidentally breathed in.

Finally, help get the victim to a doctor's office or hospital emergency room by car, ambulance, or aid car. There X-rays can be taken to show which bones (if any) are broken and where, how badly the fragments are displaced (out of normal position), whether the fracture is simple (with just two fragments) or complex (with many fragments), and other things the doctor needs to know to plan proper treatment.

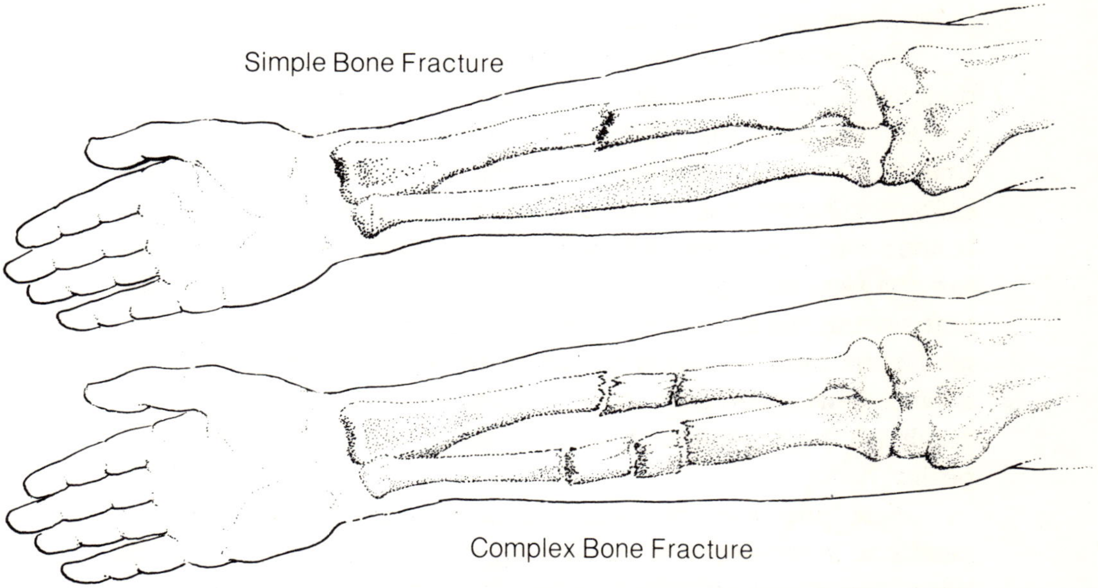

THE MIRACLE OF BONE HEALING

A broken bone must have a doctor's care, but no doctor ever healed a fracture. The *body* heals the fracture through a fascinating process of self-repair. All the doctor does is arrange things so the body can work as swiftly and perfectly as possible. So before talking about what the doctor does, let's see how the body's own natural healing process works.

Whenever a bone is broken, there is always bleeding around the break. Within just a few minutes, the blood around the fracture forms a sticky, jellylike mass that doctors call a clot, or hematoma (from Greek words meaning, literally, "lump of blood").

This hematoma has no more strength than a spoonful of Jell-O, but it forms a sort of bridge across the fractured area of bone. Within twenty-four hours, this bridge has been invaded by the two special kinds of cells we met earlier, the osteoclasts and the osteoblasts.

The osteoclasts begin work at the fracture line, slowly dissolving and reabsorbing the bone on either side of the break. This dulls the sharp edges of broken bone. At the same time the osteoblasts begin building a network of new bone cells throughout the hematoma from one side of the fracture to the other. Since these new cells contain no calcium yet, they are not very strong. But as more and more are laid down, the soft hematoma is reabsorbed by the body, and the bridge of new bone cells between the bone ends grows stronger. Even after several weeks, however, it could still be torn apart very easily, so the bone ends must be held perfectly still during this period.

How long does this first step take? It could take from two weeks to three months, depending on the size of the broken bone, the distance between the broken ends, and the total area of the fracture. The process is also much faster in the young child and slower in adults, with teenagers in between. In an elderly person, it may be very slow indeed. But it progresses just the same, until presently the broken ends of bone are glued together quite firmly by the bridge of tender new bone cells.

In the next step, the body begins to deposit calcium in the new bone cells bridging the fracture. As the calcium increases, the bridge of new bone becomes harder and stronger. Usually, this bridge is larger in diameter than the original bone and appears on an X-ray like an olive-shaped bulge around the fracture. This calcium-rich new bone is sometimes called callus. At first it is soft and chalky, but as time passes (anywhere from three weeks to three months or more, depending upon the kind of fracture and the age of the person), it gradually becomes harder and stronger until finally it is just as strong as, or stronger than, the original bone before the fracture. At this point in the healing process, it becomes safe for the victim to cautiously begin using the broken limb again.

The final step in bone healing takes place over a period of years. Slowly the new bone that has formed becomes stronger and more dense. At the same time excess new bone that was formed is gradually dissolved away by the osteoclasts. This "clean-up work" is often performed so perfectly that within a matter of two or three years it is completely impossible to tell on an X-ray film where the fracture occurred.

THE DOCTOR IN THE PICTURE

If the body heals bone so well, why do we need a doctor to help? The answer is that fractures heal best under certain special conditions. Healing is faster, for example, if the fractured bone ends are in what doctors call anatomical position —that is, very close to the unbroken bone's normal position. In addition, the healing is most perfect when the bone ends are held absolutely motionless, when there is no overlapping of fractured bones, and when no infection is present.

Unfortunately, most fractures don't come that way. Broken bone ends are often widely separated, overlapping, or sometimes even broken into fragments. Muscles near the fracture cramp and pull the fragments out of the best position for perfect healing. Thus, nature needs a doctor's help, first to set or reduce the fracture (which means, simply, manipulating it until the broken bones are in their normal position), and second, to hold the fracture fragments where they belong so they can't slip out of position again as the healing begins. Sometimes setting a fracture and holding it in proper position can be done by the family doctor. But very often the job is turned over to a bone specialist known as an orthopedist or orthopedic surgeon. Many people nowadays go directly to an orthopedist for the care of any fracture.

There are two common ways that fractures are set today. Sometimes the doctor can simply pull on the fractured limb and manipulate the bone ends into the proper position after giving the patient drugs to prevent pain. Then the entire area, from the joint below the fracture to the joint above it, is encased in a plaster cast. When this is possible without surgery, it is called a closed reduction.

More complicated fractures may require an open, or surgical, reduction. This is done when the doctor needs to use metal plates, pins, screws, or nails to hold the fracture in healing position. Once the bone fragments have been fixed (that is, held in position) in this way, the surgical opening is closed, and a plaster cast is then applied for additional support.

Infection may be a danger, especially in an open fracture (a break in which one of the broken bone ends has pierced the skin). In such a case, the doctor must clean the wound thoroughly and prescribe antibiotic medicine to help prevent bone infection later.

Once the fracture has been set and then fixed in position with a cast, the doctor will follow the healing with occasional X-rays. It's a long, boring wait for most people, hampered by a heavy plaster cast or maybe even confined to bed if a hip or thigh is broken. But it can't be helped nor hurried. Finally, the time will come—maybe two months for a fractured finger or as much as six months for a fractured thigh—when X-rays show new bone at full strength and the cast can come off. All that remains then is the slow process of getting stiff joints and weakened muscles working again before full function is restored and the fracture is healed.

SOME COMMON KINDS OF FRACTURES

There are some 206 bones in the human body, and any one of them can be broken. But for active young people, a few particular fractures are by far the most likely to occur. Most of these are related to some sport activity.

☐ *Colles fracture of the wrist.* This may be the most frequent fracture of all. It occurs when a person slips and falls, catching him- or herself on an outstretched hand. The ends of the two long bones of the forearm (the ulna and radius) are snapped off next to the wrist and shoved backward. This, in effect, pushes the whole wrist and hand back in the

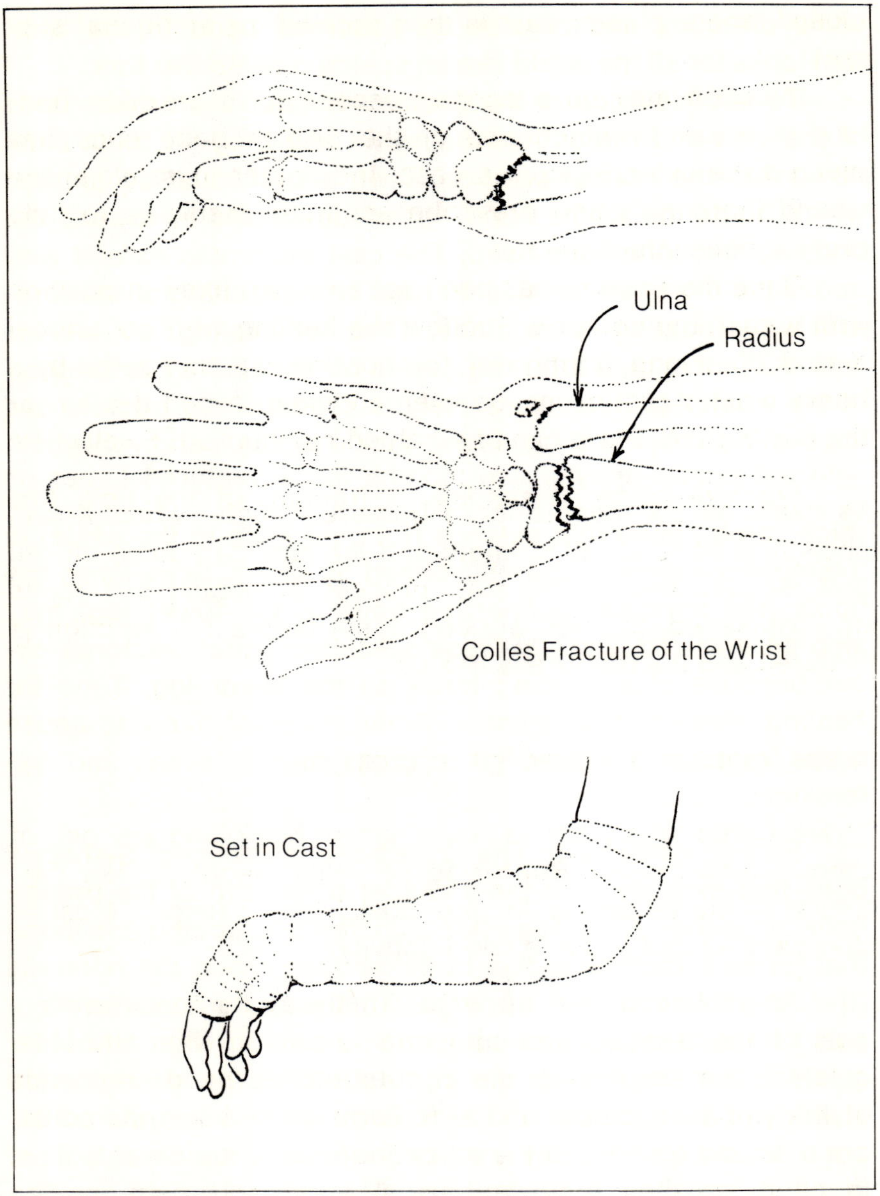

Colles Fracture of the Wrist

same direction and creates an abnormal bend in the wrist that looks for all the world like an upside down silver fork.

To set this fracture the doctor must pull the broken ends of the ulna and radius forward again and then tilt them back down into the normal position. Then a cast must be applied which holds the whole hand tipped down and in toward the body so the bones can't slip. The cast must also extend well above the elbow so there is no rotation or twisting of the forearm while healing takes place. Time for healing: six weeks, with additional time after the cast is off to restore full function of the wrist. Activities most likely to produce this fracture are ice skating, roller skating, skiing, tackle football, and volleyball.

☐ *Fracture of the lower leg.* A fracture of the tibia (the thick, strong bone that extends from the knee to the ankle) is the most common fracture sustained by skiers. Sometimes the fibula (the narrower supporting bone in the lower leg) may also be involved. Usually these so-called spiral fractures occur because of a twisting force on the lower leg. Time for healing: three to four months. Activities most likely to cause these fractures are downhill or cross-country skiing and waterskiing.

☐ *Broken collarbone.* The collarbone is the long, S-shaped bone that extends from the shoulder to the top of the breastbone on either side. Together with the shoulder blade bone that forms a shallow socket in the shoulder, and the humerus (the long bone of the upper arm), the collarbone forms a part of the three-legged structure known as the "shoulder girdle." The shoulder girdle contributes to the strength and stability of the shoulder and arm. Fortunately, when the collarbone is broken, it may not be seriously knocked out of place. It can often be drawn back into normal healing position

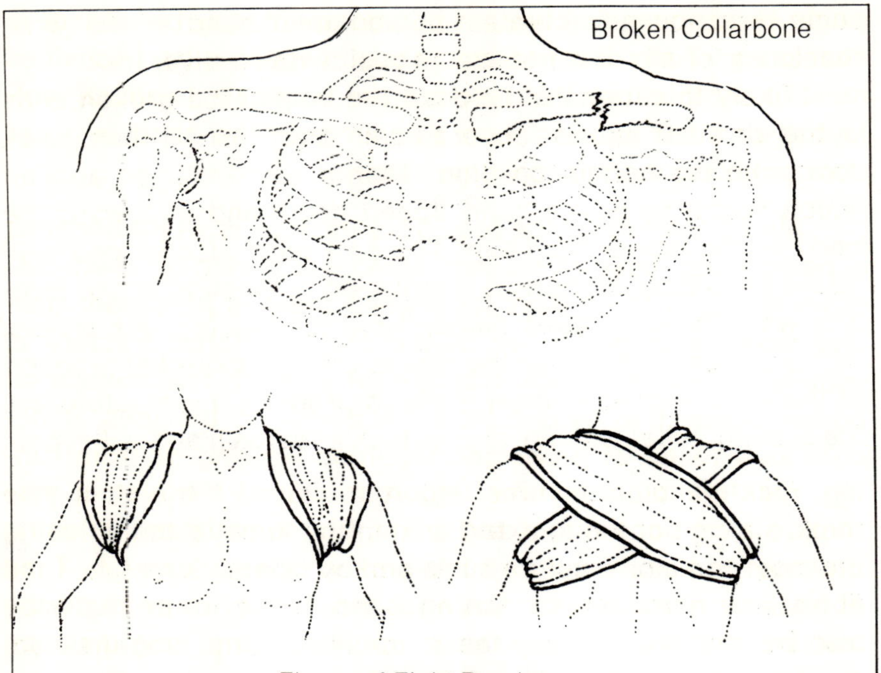

Figure-of-Eight Bandage

with a tight elastic figure-of-eight bandage wrapped under the arm and crisscrossed across the back to pull the shoulders back sharply. The time for healing: about six weeks, wearing a figure-of-eight bandage. Activities most likely to cause this fracture are tackle football and soccer.

☐ *Fractures of a finger, thumb, or hand.* The fracture may involve the fingers, thumb, or the metacarpal bones you can feel at the base of the thumb and the back of the hand. Treatment depends upon the nature of the fracture. In some cases the whole hand must be placed in a cast with a built-in traction, or pull, on the fractured bone. In other cases (such as a single finger-bone fracture), a curved splint may be all that is necessary. Time for healing: about two months. Activities most likely to cause this fracture are baseball, handball, volleyball or other injuries such as slamming the hand in a car door or hitting the thumb with a hammer.

☐ *March fracture of the foot.* This fracture is weird because a person can have it happen without knowing it, then discover it two or three days later when there is persistent pain and swelling over the top of the foot. A march fracture is usually a hairline crack fracture of one of the metatarsal bones, bones that extend from the ankles to the toes. It occurs as a result of prolonged vigorous walking or from running, rock climbing, or other vigorous use of the feet. It may require a cast of the foot and ankle. But sometimes just using crutches to keep weight off the broken bone is enough. Time of healing: a few weeks. Activities most likely to produce the fracture are hiking, track team sprinting, and long-distance running—especially early in the season when the runner is not yet in condition.

☐ *Fractures of the neck or spine.* These fractures often occur as a result of auto accidents, falls from heights, trampoline accidents, and—above all—diving accidents in which a person either bends his or her neck back too sharply on striking the water or strikes an unexpected submerged object with the head. Fractures to these bones are extremely dangerous because of possible damage to the spinal cord. See special first-aid precautions discussed earlier.

CHAPTER 4

JOINT DISLOCATIONS

Dislocation of a joint is quite a different sort of injury from a fracture. For one thing, when a joint is dislocated, there are not usually any broken bones involved. This means the victim may not have the long period of healing so often necessary for fractures. What is more, dislocations occur more rarely than fractures. But dislocations and fractures do have certain things in common. Both are usually the result of sudden blows, falls, or other violent injuries to the body. Both are often associated with active sports. Both are extremely painful when they occur, and, until they have received proper medical treatment, both severely limit the motion and function of the involved part.

What is a dislocation? It is an injury in which the bones in a joint are pulled or knocked out of position so that the joint surfaces are no longer in contact. Because each of our joints is surrounded by a tough envelope of fibrous tissue helping to hold it together, a dislocation almost always means tearing of the joint capsule too. It also means bleeding into the joint and, in some cases, it may cause severe stretching or other damage to important nerves and blood vessels in the area.

Thus, a dislocation is a serious injury. It requires proper treatment and enough time for healing around the joint so that the dislocation will not tend to happen again later.

FIRST AID FOR DISLOCATIONS

Because the symptoms are so very much the same, you may not be able to tell a dislocation from a fracture. But the basic principles of first aid are exactly the same as discussed earlier. In addition, with a possible dislocation victim, every effort should be made to get help to the patient or to get the patient to an emergency room as quickly as possible, especially if the injury seems to affect the motion of a shoulder or a hip. The reason is that when a dislocation occurs, circulation of blood to the limb may be sharply decreased or even cut off. The sooner the bones are returned to the right position, the better the chances of recovery without any serious blood vessel or nerve injury.

HOW DISLOCATIONS ARE TREATED

The doctor's first job is to get the misplaced bones back into their natural position in the joint with as little additional injury or damage as possible. This is called reducing the dislocation. To do this, the doctor must first find out exactly where the misplaced bones are in relation to each other. X-rays will help tell this and will also show if there is any fracture of the bone—a rather uncommon but serious complication of a dislocation.

To reduce the dislocation, the doctor may first administer some medicine to relieve pain and help the victim relax (muscles may be cramping in the area surrounding the dislocation). Then the dislocation is reduced by pulling and manipulating the bones until they are properly replaced in the joint. When a huge, powerful joint such as the hip is dislocated, general anesthesia may be necessary for sufficient relaxation to allow the reduction.

Once the bone is back in its proper place, the doctor will use either a plaster cast or a firm elastic wrapper to hold the reduced joint still and prevent the victim from moving it. The joint must be fixed, or held still in this fashion long enough for the swelling in and about the joint to go down and long enough for the torn joint capsule to heal. For a finger joint, which must be moved early to prevent stiffness, this may be a period of a few days followed by four to six weeks of protective splinting. For a shoulder or a hip, the time of protection may extend to a couple of months or more.

COMMON DISLOCATIONS

Here are some of the more frequent dislocations that occur in young people.

☐ *Dislocated finger.* This injury most often occurs as a result of attempting to catch a baseball without a glove—so frequently, in fact, that it is sometimes called "baseball finger." It can also occur to volleyball players. A blow from the flying ball striking the finger end-on simply pushes the finger bone back out of joint. There is considerable pain, the tip

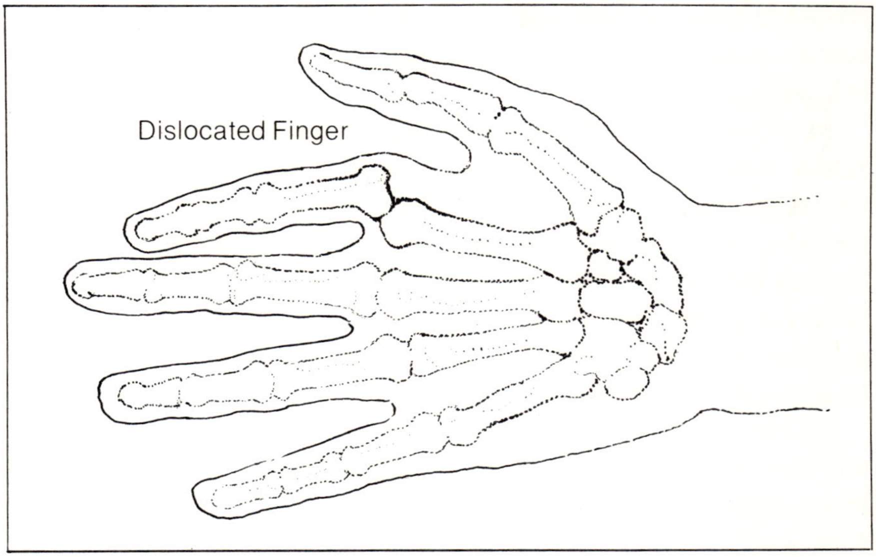

of the finger will no longer move, and the deformity is hard to miss.

This is one of the simplest of dislocations to treat. The doctor simply pulls on the tip of the finger until the joint pops back into position. This usually relieves most of the pain and restores movement to the finger. All the same, an X-ray may be taken to be sure a piece of bone has not been chipped off. Once a finger dislocation has been reduced, the finger is usually held motionless with a curved splint and kept bandaged for a period of four to six weeks.

☐ *Dislocated jaw.* This injury occasionally occurs during vigorous contact sports such as football, boxing, or wrestling. Most often, however, it happens as a result (believe it or not) of over-vigorous yawning. The hinge of the jaw pops out

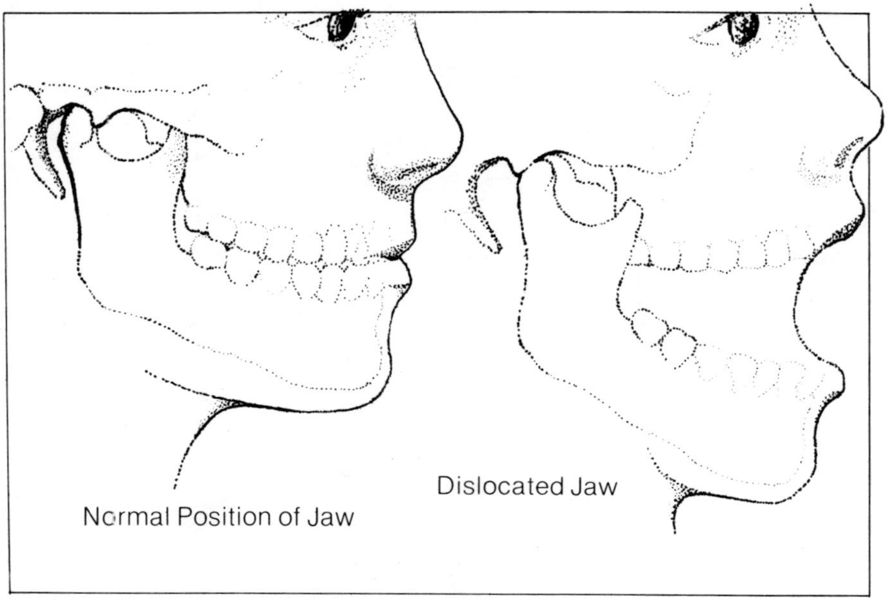

of joint when the mouth is opened too widely, locking the jaw wide open. To reduce this dislocation the doctor pads both of his or her thumbs thoroughly with gauze, grasps the lower jaw firmly with the thumbs flat against the rear molar teeth, and then pushes downward and backward until the jaw goes back into place. (The padding is needed because the jaw closes with a snap the moment the dislocation is reduced!) As long as no bone is broken, no further treatment is needed except, possibly, some aspirin; the hinge of the jaw on either side will be sore for several days.

□ *Dislocation of the shoulder.* This striking injury can result from falls, vigorous or body contact sports, or anything else that exerts an extreme and unnatural force upon the

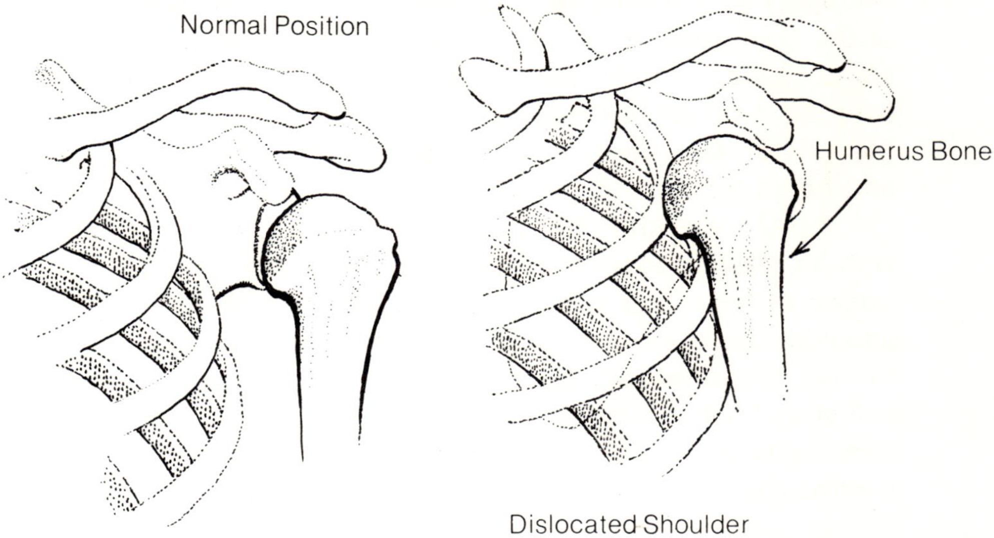

shoulder. It is especially distressing to the victim because it looks and feels absolutely awful. There is extreme pain in the shoulder, with numbness and tingling extending down the arm to the wrist, hand, or fingers. The normal roundness at the point of the shoulder is replaced by a flatness or even a hollow, and one can often feel the head of the humerus bone —the large bone of the upper arm—jammed down into the armpit where it obviously doesn't belong. Finally, the arm will be held at an awkward angle and the victim will be unable to move it or use it.

In treating this dislocation the doctor will first use some medicine to relieve the pain and help relax muscles. Then, with the patient lying on his or her stomach on an examining table with the dislocated shoulder over the edge, the doctor will apply gentle traction and manipulation to place the head of the bone into its socket again. This may also be done, in some cases, with the patient sitting in a chair with the arm over the back of it. Once the dislocation has been reduced, the doctor will check to be certain that both circulation and nerve function to the arm and hand have been restored.

Finally, the arm and forearm will be bound to the chest with an elastic binder to prevent motion of the shoulder for a period of time. This is especially important with a dislocated shoulder because the dislocation may tear a hole in the fibrous capsule around the joint. Unless that hole is given sufficient time to heal closed, the victim may well have recurrent dislocations, making it necessary for a surgeon to open the shoulder and sew the torn capsule shut again.

☐ *Dislocation of the hip.* The ball-and-socket joint of the hip, surrounded by powerful muscles and tough ligaments, is one of the largest and strongest joints in the body. Thus, it can be dislocated only by the most extreme violence—in an automobile collision, for example, or falling out of a tree. When dislocation does occur, usually the ball of the femur is jarred out of place to the rear, and the thigh is bent outward and cannot be moved. The dislocation is extremely painful and may often involve a fracture of the thighbone or the pelvis as well.

Reduction of such a dislocation usually requires a general anesthetic in order to relax cramped muscles sufficiently to get the bone back into proper position. After reduction the pelvis and leg may be placed in a plaster cast or in traction to hold the hip joint motionless until the fibrous capsule of the hip and other supporting ligaments have time to heal. This could mean anywhere from several weeks to several months, depending upon how much other damage has been done to the joint.

☐ *Dislocations Which Aren't Dislocations.* Sometimes painful muscular or skeletal conditions are thought to be dislocations but don't really involve any dislocation at all. One of these conditions is wry neck, or torticollis. This is a sharp muscular pain that occurs in the neck and shoulder, usually on one side, so that the victim cannot comfortably turn his or her head. It may *feel* as though a bone in the neck has slipped out of place, but nothing of the sort has happened. Wry neck is purely a matter of painful muscle spasm, often related to nervous tension, exhaustion, or exposure to cold and damp. It can be relieved best with rest and the application of hot moist towels to the area until the pain goes away.

Some people are afflicted with similar severe pain in the middle or lower back, usually after bending over to lift some heavy load without bending their knees. It feels as if they have "thrown out their back"—but again, it is a matter of painful muscle spasm and not any bone dislocation. After all, the vertebrae are solid, chunky pieces of bone that are tightly bound together with ligaments and are, under ordinary circumstances, practically impossible to dislocate.

Still other people speak of "throwing out their sacroiliac." They are referring to the long, flat joint between the sacrum (the bone at the base of the spine) and the adjoining portion of the pelvic bone known as the iliac segment. This sacroiliac joint is bound tightly by ligaments and tendons and is rarely, if ever, actually dislocated. Rather, irritation of that joint can cause a painful muscle spasm in the lower back and buttocks which may require rest, heat, and muscle-relaxing medicines for treatment.

Occasionally, when a bone is dislocated, a fracture may also occur. This is a major complication and always makes the treatment more difficult. First, of course, the dislocated bone must be replaced in its proper position. But after that, the doctor is basically treating a fracture, not a dislocation, and will treat it like any other fracture.

CHAPTER 5

SPRAINS AND STRAINS

Just as dislocations are usually less serious injuries than fractures, sprains and strains of joints are generally less serious than dislocations. They are certainly painful enough and need proper treatment. But usually they take less time to heal and are less likely to cause long-term trouble and disability.

People use the words sprain and strain as if they meant the same thing, but they are really two somewhat different injuries. A *sprain* occurs when a joint has been twisted or wrenched so severely that some of the supporting ligaments of the joint have been torn. This means that these ligaments must heal before the joint regains its full strength and stability. A *strain* occurs when a muscle, or a tendon connected to a muscle has been pulled, bruised, or torn. (This may occur in the vicinity of a joint, but not always; a muscle in the thigh or back, for example, can be strained.)

Generally, but not always, a sprain of a joint will be a more serious injury than a strain and will take longer to heal. When a joint is sprained there will be pain and swelling in the area, which tends to settle down fairly quickly as long as you don't continue using the injured joint. There will also be internal bleeding. This may show up later as black-and-blue marks appearing on the skin. First-aid treatment consists of applying a pressure dressing to the injured joint, preferably with an elastic bandage; elevation of the injured area, whenever this is possible; and strict nonuse of the joint for the first twenty-four hours. If pain or swelling persists longer than that, the sprain may be severe and should be examined by a doctor, who will take X-rays to be sure no fracture has occurred and then prescribe the proper treatment to allow the sprain to heal.

SOME COMMON SPRAINS

A sprained ankle is probably the most frequently occurring sprain of all. This is hardly surprising. Each of your ankles has a tough job to do, supporting the full weight of your body alternately with the other whenever you stand, walk, or run. Yet the ankle is not very strong or stable, as joints go. It must depend heavily on a tight binding of ligaments and tendons to keep it in place. Of all the joints, it is the one most likely to be twisted or wrenched—and this shows up in the frequency with which doctors must treat sprained ankles.

Probably the next most frequent sprain—suffered by almost everyone at one time or another—is a sprained thumb. Sometimes it is the first joint of the thumb (right at the V between the thumb and the first finger) that is sprained. At other times it is the joint farther back, connecting the thumb with the wrist. In either case the sprain can cause a marked swelling of the thumb and part of the hand; it may also hurt severely and turn an ugly black-and-blue color. Such a sprain requires a doctor's attention. In some cases it may be enough to hold the thumb still with a splint and elastic wrapper, protected from further injury, until healing has taken place—usually an interval of seven to fourteen days. But some kinds of thumb sprains require surgery.

Next to the thumb, the little finger of the hand is most likely to be sprained, partly because it is the weakest of the fingers and partly because it is the finger that can be separated most widely from the others. However, any joint of any of the fingers can be sprained. Recovery from finger sprains is usually much quicker than from a severe sprain of the thumb.

A sprain of the wrist can occur when you fall on an outstretched hand hard enough to wrench the wrist but not hard enough to cause a fracture. To treat a wrist sprain a specially molded plastic splint is often useful, extending from the palm back along the forearm, and held in place by an elastic bandage. This leaves the fingers and thumb free to move but prevents motion of the wrist until the sprain has healed.

Occasionally a baseball pitcher suffers an injury to the shoulder of his or her pitching arm as a result of its overuse. This injury involves a tearing of some of the muscle fibers that cross the shoulder and allow the arm its wide range of motion. Doctors suspect it when the player's shoulder becomes sore and he or she has difficulty raising the pitching arm up above shoulder level. Fortunately, this injury is far more common among professional baseball players who pitch often, than among those playing amateur ball.

One other sprain-type injury often heard about but seldom seen in young people is a special kind of sprain of the knee that occurs among professional football and basketball players. The knee is a heavy, solid, weight-bearing joint, second only to the hip in the amount of work it must do. Yet because it is a simple hinge joint, it is not terribly strong, especially when it is twisted under pressure. Some protection from twisting is provided by special crescent-shaped pieces of cartilage that lie on either side of the knee, the so-called semilunar cartilages, and by special supporting ligaments called collateral ligaments. Unfortunately, in the extreme rough-and-tumble of professional football or basketball, a player's semilunar cartilages or collateral ligaments, or both, may be torn. The result is an unstable and painful knee. Sometimes this kind of injury will heal by itself, in time, if the player's knee is properly strapped and the player is taken off the playing field for a season. But if the injury recurs, it may be necessary to have the torn structures treated by surgery.

PREVENTING FRACTURES, DISLOCATIONS, AND SPRAINS

Everyone would agree that none of these injuries is pleasant to have happen. All of them cause pain. All of them require the victim to stop using some important part of the body for a while—sometimes quite a long while. Certainly it would be desirable to prevent such injuries if there were any way to do it. And, to some degree, they *can* be prevented.

Of course there are always accidents that no one can foresee or prevent. Nevertheless, attention to a few simple rules can considerably reduce the number of fractures, dislocations, and sprains.

(1) Try to be in top physical shape for the kind of physical activity you want to undertake. The person who has no physical exercise, to speak of, all winter and spring and then takes a 12-mile (19 km) hike in the mountains the first day school is out, is begging for trouble. A regular program of year-round sports activity will help you keep in physical shape. Even if you aren't interested in organized sports, a regular program of physical exercise such as jogging, bicycling, tennis, or swimming will strengthen your muscles, improve your coordination, build stronger joints, and make it far less likely you will experience bone and joint injuries.

(2) Know your sport, its rules, its demands, and its requirements. Try to obtain and use good equipment for the kind of activity you are going to engage in. For hiking or rock scrambling, get a good sturdy pair of hiking boots that provide firm support for your ankles; don't start up the trail in a pair of tennis shoes. If you are going to play baseball, obtain and use a proper mitt (as well as a hard hat when you are up to bat). If you want to ski, see that you're dressed properly for the weather. Also see to it that you have a good pair of ski boots that provide support to your ankles, and be sure the safety bindings on your skis actually work. Snowmobilers should make a habit of operating their machines from a standing or kneeling position, not sitting—sitting snowmobilers have been known to crush vertebrae in their lower backs from unexpected impacts. Football players should not only wear the customary protective gear but should also keep their ankles and knees properly taped for support until they are in top physical condition. Protective sports equipment

has been developed over the years for the sole purpose of *protecting,* usually against fractures, dislocations, and sprains. It doesn't make sense not to use such equipment.

(3) Anticipate trouble, and keep an eye out for it at all times. This is simply a matter of habit and common sense. If you see ice on a flight of stairs, get a good grip on the handrail before you start down. Late in the day, when you are hiking downhill and almost exhausted, slow your pace down, and make sure of your footing with each step. This is the time when hikers sprain ankles or break legs. There are dozens of other common-sense ways you can foresee possible trouble in one activity or another and either avoid it or be mentally prepared in advance to deal with it. Common sense can tell you that trampolines are deadly devices that can snap necks, just as common sense should tell you not to take a running dive into an unknown body of water.

This is not to say that you must be timid and fearful about everything you do—far from it. All we're talking about is staying alert and using common sense. There is nothing particularly courageous about taking unnecessary risks with the only body you will ever have. Develop your ability to recognize danger in advance, and use common sense to avoid injuries whenever possible. The bones you save may be your own.

GLOSSARY

BONE—The hard, calcium-filled tissue that makes up the 200-plus bones that give our bodies their shape and strength. Although it appears "dead," bone is actually very much a living tissue. (See TISSUE)

CARTILAGE—A soft, glossy, slippery tissue that coats the ends of bones where they meet in joints. Cartilage contains little calcium. In infants the bones are mostly cartilage before calcium is deposited to make them hard and strong.

CAPSULE—The envelope or wrapper of tough fibers that surround and support movable joints in the body.

DISLOCATION—A tearing or jarring apart of the bones of a joint, so that the joint no longer fits or functions.

FIBROUS TISSUE—A tissue made up of tough, stringy strands or fibers, sometimes in layers. Fibrous tissue may provide strength and support to a part of the body, or it may *connect* one part of the body to another firmly.

FRACTURE—Any break in a bone. In a SIMPLE FRACTURE, the break is in a single line. In a COMPLEX FRACTURE, the break involves several to many fragments (as when a portion of bone is crushed). In a CLOSED FRACTURE, none of the broken bone fragments pierce the skin. In an OPEN FRACTURE, one or more bone fragments have broken through the skin.

JOINT—Any place where two or more bones meet. At a MOVABLE JOINT (knee, elbow, etc.), the joint is constructed to permit movement. In a FIXED JOINT (skull bones, pelvic bones), no motion is intended.

LIGAMENT—A thick, tough strap or rope of fibrous tissue. Many joints are surrounded by ligaments to give them strength and support.

MARROW—The substances found in the interior cavities of bones. YELLOW MARROW is largely fat and is found in the hollow shafts of long bones. RED MARROW is found inside the bulging ends of bones and produces many of the body's blood cells.

MUSCLE—The soft, meaty tissue that makes up much of the bulk of the body. Muscle has the power to *contract* and *pull;* when it is attached to bone, it can pull the bone, thus permitting movement of the body.

OSTEOBLASTS—"Bone-building" cells which produce new bone cells and permit them to be filled with calcium and phosphorous compounds. They are important in replacement of bone cells to heal over a fracture.

OSTEOCLASTS—"Bone-destroying" cells which dissolve calcium from bone cells. They work in partnership with osteoblasts to get rid of old or damaged bone so that new bone can be built.

REDUCTION—The mechanical replacement of a broken bone or dislocated joint to its original (uninjured), normal position. Necessary for healing to take place.

SPRAIN—A twisting or wrenching injury to a joint in which the supporting ligaments or capsule or fibrous tissue is torn or damaged.

STRAIN—A twisting or wrenching injury, often but not always to a joint, in which a muscle or tendon is pulled or torn.

TENDON—A strip of tough fibrous tissue that emerges from the end of a muscle. A muscle is usually attached to a bone by means of a tendon.

TISSUE—Any group of cells that forms a part of the body.

ADDITIONAL READING

Abramson, Seth F., M.D., and Schultz, Dodi. *Home and Family Emergencies.* Des Moines: Meredith, 1973.

American College of Surgeons, Committee on Trauma; Kennedy, Robert H., M.D., ed. *Emergency Care of the Sick and Injured,* pp. 66—72. Philadelphia: W. B. Saunders, 1966.

Asimov, Isaac. *The Human Body.* pp. 27—119. Boston: Houghton Mifflin, 1963.

Nourse, Alan E., and the editors of *Life. The Body.* pp. 54—75. New York: Time Inc., 1964.

Red Cross, U.S. American National Red Cross. *Standard First Aid and Personal Safety.* pp. 18—65, 195—224, 225—253. New York: Doubleday, 1973.

INDEX

ABOUT THE AUTHOR

Alan Nourse is a former practicing physician and a well-known science writer. For Franklin Watts, he has written the acclaimed *Lumps, Bumps, and Rashes: A Look at Kids' Diseases* and *Viruses* for the First Book series. One of Dr. Nourse's favorite hobbies is astronomy, and he has written many books for Franklin Watts on the subject, including *The Backyard Astronomer.*